SMARTER MEDICINE

HOW
ARTIFICIAL
INTELLIGENCE
WILL MAKE YOU
HEALTHIER

YOUSIF A-RAHIM, MD, PhD

Lecturer in Medicine, Harvard Medical School
Chief Medical Officer at Covenant Physician Partners

Boston, MA USA

For my parents,
who made my future the purpose of their lives

The future of Well-Being will be precise, personalized, predictable, participatory, and process oriented. AI and deep learning AI-generated ecosystems of self-regulation and bioregulation through digiceuticals are the next frontiers. The book you hold in your hands is prescient.

-Deepak Chopra, MD, The Chopra Foundation, DeepakChopra.com

Smarter Medicine is a rhapsody of powerful wisdom that illustrates how machine learning can bring greater humanity to health care. Harvard physician Dr. A-Rahim takes us on a thrilling adventure deep into the world of artificial intelligence and a future where AI works in partnership with physicians to augment their knowledge, safeguard against misdiagnosis and medication errors, reduce health care costs, and perhaps most importantly, rapidly detect disease
at a point when it is most curable.
This intelligent pageturner is a resource for both physicians and non-physicians; literally, it is for anyone with an interest in medicine and curiosity about it can adapt to create a healthier world. It spills over with compelling anecdotes, history, and examples of how AI can revolutionize specialties ranging from pathology to cardiology, mental health, gastroenterology, radiology, and robotic surgery, and over time make you and your family healthier. As Dr. A-Rahim suggests,
AI does not replace doctors but has the potential to
eplace those doctors who do not use its gifts.

-Gina Vild, co-author of The Two Most Important Days, How to Find your Purpose and Live a Happier, Healthier Life, and past Associate Dean and Chief Communications Officer at Harvard Medical School

Artificial intelligence has the potential to transform the practice of medicine for clinicians and patients. Smarter Medicine provides an intriguing look at the many ways in which the application of AI is already improving diagnosis and treatment across a range of medical specialties. The potential implications of AI on patient outcomes and health equity presented in this book will make you hopeful and excited for the future of healthcare.

-Max Lin, KKR Partner and leader of KKR's Americas Private Equity platform

Dr. A-Rahim provides an articulate, brilliant, and captivating overview of artificial intelligence's potential to transform how we diagnose and treat common maladies afflicting humans. He discusses how AI can be used to develop better diagnostic tools, identify risk factors for diseases, predict outcomes for patients, and much more. In addition, he highlights the potential benefits that AI could bring to underserved populations worldwide who often lack access to quality healthcare.

The implications of this book are far-reaching and will alter how we view disease, health, and health equity—a must-read for anyone interested in the future of healthcare.

-Sanjiv Chopra MD MACP FRCP, Professor of Medicine, Harvard Medical School.

Dr. A-Rahim presents a very compelling and timely argument for the advanced use of AI in medicine. Dr. A highlights several specialties where advanced use of AI would bring immediate benefits to better patient outcomes, higher patient satisfaction, and lower system cost. Due to the charm and wit of the author, the material is presented in an easy-to-consume manner. This book is an essential read for physicians and lay persons alike.

-Lew Little, Jr., Executive Chairman and Board Chair, EQ Health Acquisition, former Chief Executive Officer of Harden Healthcare

Dr. A-Rahim's book provides insight into how Artificial Intelligence is used today in healthcare. It also provides a futuristic view of how medicine will be practiced and patients will be diagnosed and treated. It's a must-read book for physicians, nurses, health care executives, and anyone interested in the potential of artificial intelligence to transform health care worldwide.

-Wendy Arnone, Independent Board Member and Retired Healthcare Executive with over 35 years of experience in the healthcare industry

Artificial intelligence has been a reality in medicine for quite some time now. Dr. A-Rahim vividly illustrates how AI has already begun to change and improve medical care. He also makes a strong case for why AI will become even more critical in the future as our population continues to grow and age.

-Mohamed Abdelrahim, GM, Jubaili Holdings Dubai, UAE

TABLE OF CONTENTS

PREFACE

I am a Harvard-trained practicing physician, a scientist, and a health-care executive who believes in artificial intelligence's revolutionary and transformative power in medicine. With artificial intelligence, we can detect diseases earlier, provide more accurate diagnoses and treatments, and even cure diseases; the future of medicine lies in artificial intelligence.

In December 2021, I was invited to give a keynote speech on artificial intelligence in medicine at the prestigious Harvard Continuing Medical Education course for Internal Medicine. Delivering a keynote at Harvard was a huge honor, and my primary goal was not to embarrass myself! Fortunately, the talk was extremely well received, and it sparked a lively discussion and numerous questions during the Q&A. Within an hour of finishing the talk, my phone started buzzing with messages from the course director, Dr. Sanjiv Chopra, professor and former Dean at Harvard Medical School, complimenting me on my talk. "You did a great job!" he exclaimed. "Now, you need to write a book about the topic. You've already done the research!"

I rose from my desk upon reading Dr. Chopra's missives. "Are you kidding me?" I yelled out loud in disbelief that he was serious about me writing a book on artificial intelligence. Indeed, I thought Sanjiv was generous with his feedback; he is one of the sweetest people. But then, Sanjiv is never one to mince words either; he is always direct with his positive and negative feedback. "You are too kind!" was all I could think of in reply. But then he followed up with an ultimatum: "I will give you 30 days to do it, and if you are too busy, then I expect it in 28 days!"

I was honored by Dr. Chopra's suggestion and quickly realized that it was hard to argue with him. After all, he is a world-renowned physician and author with an uncanny ability to get what he wants.

That was the pregnant moment that gave birth to this modest project. It was flattering but also daunting. I embarked on this undertaking with a bit of trepidation and excitement. It has been a fantastic experience: one I will never forget. Of course, the book took well over 28 days to write.

This book is about the computer revolution in medicine. It is written for clinicians, computer scientists, and students of medicine, nursing, and computer science, as well as the lay public. I believe primary care practitioners have much to gain from reading this book. Primary care is the hero's profession and the backbone of our healthcare system. Primary care is where most patients receive their care, and many critical decisions about a patient's health are made; it is poised to benefit the most from advances in computer science.

I have been a physician for nearly 25 years and have seen firsthand how technology has changed healthcare. I remember when we started using computers to chart our patients' visits; it was a vast improvement over writing everything by hand. We could better track our patients' progress over time and see patterns we couldn't see before. Alas, the electronic health care record has now become why some of us want to bolt and run away from medicine.

This book focuses on the artificial intelligence applications that are changing medicine and some of the opportunities and challenges of this change. In my research, I have found that artificial intelligence has already begun to revolutionize healthcare in many ways. For example, it improves patient care by helping doctors make better decisions, reduce diagnostic errors, speed up medical diagnoses, and provide personalized treatments for patients. Revolutionary and transformative, artificial intelligence can help us do our jobs better by providing us with more information at our fingertips and keeping us up to date on all aspects of medicine. This technology empowers us to provide better quality care to our patients because we have more timely information when making decisions about their treatment plans.

However, some challenges are associated with implementing artificial intelligence into clinical practice, such as ensuring that data is accurate and secure, integrating the technology into existing clinical workflows, and training the workforce to use it effectively. Other concerns need to be addressed as well. For example, there is a risk that patients could be over-diagnosed or over-treated if they receive care from machines rather than human doctors. There is also the possibility that data collected by machines could be used for nefarious purposes like identity theft or insurance fraud.

The potential for artificial intelligence in medicine is limitless, and I believe it will play an increasingly important role in our healthcare system over the next few years. EVERY clinician needs to be aware of artificial intelligence's potential paradigm shift in medicine. I am excited to see where this technology takes us and look forward to its impact on patient care.

Science is naturally cumulative. Every discovery builds on what has come before. This book is a heavily researched piece of work. I have used a variety of sources to compile it, including online research, scholarly journals, and books. I have extensively drawn on the brilliant work of others to create this book. The quality of their research is what makes my work possible. It would be impossible to name them all, but I want to express my gratitude to them nonetheless. I have cited their research throughout, and I urge you to look at it.

Yousif A-Rahim, MD, PhD
Boston, MA, USA

## CHAPTER 1

ARTIFICIAL INTELLIGENCE: THE 4THINDUSTRIAL REVOLUTION

When IBM® Deep Blue®, an artificial intelligence algorithm, defeated the world chess champion, Gary Kasparov, in 1997, it was a seminal moment in humanity's history. Kasparov was devastated. Not only did he lose to artificial intelligence (AI), but it was his first loss ever!

No human has beaten a computer in a chess tournament in nearly 17 years. Moreover, advances in AI have since made chess-playing computers even more sophisticated and formidable than the original versions. Without completely glamorizing this feat of AI and its significance in the history of our civilization, it is fair to say that for centuries we saw mastery in chess as the peak accomplishment of man's intellectual powers. In 2011, IBM Watson bested two top Jeopardy champions.

Go is arguably the most complex board game in existence. Its goal is "simple": Surround more territory than your opponent. Humans have played this game for the past 2500 years, which is thought to be the oldest board game. However, it is not only humans that are playing this game now. In 2016, Google DeepMind's AlphaGo, an AI algorithm, defeated the 18-time world Go champion Lee Sedol in four out of five games.

Usually, a computer beating a human at a game like chess or checkers would not be that impressive. But Go is different. Go cannot be solved by brute force. Go cannot be predicted. There are over 10^{170} moves possible in Go. To put that in perspective, there are only 10^{80} atoms in the observable universe.

AlphaGo was trained using data from actual human Go games. It ran through millions of rounds, learned the techniques, and even created new moves that no one had ever seen. Alone this is impressive; however, only a year after AlphaGo's victory over Lee Sedol, Google DeepMind created a brand-new AI called AlphaGo Zero, which beat the original AlphaGo. Not in four out of five games, not in five out of five games, not in ten out of ten games, but it beat AlphaGo 100 – 0, 100 games in a row. The most impressive part is that AlphaGo Zero learned to play with zero human interaction. It only played against AlphaGo, and it played millions of games. This technique was more powerful than any previous version because it was not limited to human knowledge of the game.

No data was given, no historical figures were provided, only the game's fundamental rules. AlphaGo Zero surpassed AlphaGo in just 40 days of learning. In only 40 days, AlphaGo Zero managed to best over 2500 years of strategy and knowledge, demonstrating that an AI algorithm can train to a superhuman level without human examples or expertise. AlphaGo Zero is now considered the best Go player in the world. If AI can learn how to play without human interaction, create its strategies, and beat us with those strategies, there will be more non-human knowledge about Go than humans. And if we continue to develop artificial intelligence, there will be more and more non-human intelligence. Eventually, perhaps, we reach a point where we represent a minority of intelligence, maybe even a minuscule amount.

These are exciting times for AI. When you hear the term artificial intelligence, what comes to mind? Super-powered robots? Hyper-intelligent devices? Science fiction has familiarized the world with the concept, but what is AI, and what can AI do outside Hollywood? AI involves using computers to do things that usually require human intelligence. AI is the science of making machines intelligent, using algorithms that allow computers to solve problems that used to be solved only by humans.

We all have probably dealt with AI at some point in our lives. Whether you realize it or not, AI is already all around us and is changing the world daily. The world uses AI in sports and education, music and movies, business, and news. AI powers search engines, autocorrect, email categorization, smart streaming, online shopping recommendations, and digital assistants. Enjoy streaming music and videos? When we watch films, listen to music, or shop online, AI gives us suggestions about what we might like. Streaming services like Netflix and YouTube use AI-based recommendation systems to analyze consumer interests and preferences and offer personalized recommendations.

AI is reducing the hassle of daily commuting. Another example is commuting and navigation. Whether commuting by personal car or public transport, AI – and machine learning-powered mobile apps make it simpler with real-time data on traffic routes, distance, and time.

Another ubiquitous use of AI is in voice assistance. AI voice assistants like Amazon Alexa, Google Assistant, and iPhone Siri can simplify life in highly effective ways: scheduling meetings, updating weather conditions, making appointments, or playing a requested musical number.

Another example of AI in everyday life is AI-based secure verification. Smart unlock and verification of smartphones, security systems, and other gadgets rely on AI, as does facial recognition technology, to verify and provide user access. The latter uses subsets of AI, computer vision, and machine learning.

AI technologies today are brilliant, and the possibilities endless, from fraud prevention to developing new strategies to address climate change. Astronomers use AI to find and evaluate exoplanets and distant solar systems. In the educational sector, AI helps individualize learning activities on digital platforms. Unhappy motorists are using AI (DoNotPay) to discover if they can overturn parking fines. AI can convert spoken language into text and translate it into other languages. AI is a central component of robotics. Robots make our everyday lives easier. Without AI, self-driving cars would not exist. AI enables self-driving vehicles to see and recognize their environment and react to it.

AI in medicine, the focus of this book, is another robust application of these intelligent algorithms. AI is becoming increasingly important in medicine. For instance, AI supports clinicians when diagnosing diseases and predicting responses to treatments. Radiologists can use AI to calculate tumors' exact shape and volume, revolutionizing treatment. Also, more and more patients use AI-based apps for initial diagnosis. I shall discuss in detail multiple innovative applications and examples of AI in medicine that are studied today.

AI is the future of medicine. As clinicians, once we understand how AI works, we can better gauge where it can support everyday clinical activities and decision-making. With continual enhancements in AI algorithms, AI is getting better and better at helping us; for this, we need an AI-competent community. Medicine with AI at its heart has the power to change the world. As clinicians, it is imperative that we directly engage with shaping AI development and progress in healthcare to ensure a prolific and fruitful future with AI. My deep conviction and argument, which I will lay out in the ensuing pages, is that AI is here to stay; it will not replace humans or doctors but will perhaps replace doctors who do not use AI.

## CHAPTER 2

AI DECIPHERS COMPLEX DATA

How Does AI Work?
And What Problem or Problems Does It Solve?

"We are not provided with wisdom, we must discover it for ourselves, after a journey through the wilderness..." remarked the French novelist and critic Marcel Proust. "Information is not knowledge. The only source of knowledge is an experience," is a quotation attributed to Albert Einstein, and "Experience is the best teacher" is another famous one attributed to Julius Caesar.

Learning happens best when we each experience it for ourselves in the real world. This typifies human nature and the limits of *human intelligence*. While tried and true, it is inefficient and not always practical to rely on lived experience alone to wisely live your life. For a human to become sagacious and experience everything there is to experience, they would have to live forever. In other words, become superhuman. But what if there was a practical way or a hack that allowed us to download all our historical wisdom and put it into practice right away? In other words, the opposite of what Proust, Einstein, and Caesar suggested. Become wise without having experienced it all yourself.

Well, it exists! It's called *non-human intelligence* or AI, which, unlike human intelligence, is limitless. AI has learned everything in the past. It's been at every crossroads and will *always* predict the best outcomes and pitfalls to avoid. For instance, you don't necessarily need to get lost a dozen times in San Francisco before you are shown the ropes. You can use Waze, AI-powered smart navigation. AI helps you download decades of San Francisco traffic wisdom in real-time. In an instant, you become superhuman.

AI uses the vastness of the past to predict the future. And it does so by building on potentially millions of past occurrences from which to conclude. Put simply, *past* patterns, clusters, and trends are used by powerful, intelligent algorithms in the *present* to enable a computer program to predict the *future.*

In essence, AI is inspired by the famous quotation attributed to the late Harvard philosopher Santayana: "Those who cannot remember the past are condemned to repeat it." People who don't learn from their mistakes don't mature. Couples who do not learn from their fights break up. Life is lived in the present, but its significance is appreciated in hindsight.

What exactly is artificial intelligence? We speak of AI when computer systems perform tasks that usually require human intelligence. Powered by complex algorithms, a computer program uses clusters, patterns, and trends to combine different sources of information and generate a result that essentially mimics human behavior. This includes recognizing images, making decisions, or engaging in dialogue.

To do this, the AI systems must be equipped with knowledge and experience. We can achieve this in two ways. You can program each instruction so that the machine solves the tasks step by step. This is comparable to a cooking recipe or assembly instructions. Alternatively, you can use programs that learn from the data independently. This enables these programs or algorithms to detect relevant information to draw conclusions or make predictions. This is known as machine learning. A term sometimes used to refer to AI.

Now, let's look under the hood. This chapter will explore the technology that underpins AI, what it is, how it works, and how it solves problems. I will briefly review the history of AI. I intend to be clinical: Avoid minutiae and only discuss the broad technical aspects of AI that a clinician, computer scientist, or curious layperson needs to know. For those who want a deeper dive into AI's methodology, I recommend *Artificial Intelligence: A New Synthesis* by the brilliant scientist and leading researcher Nils J. Nilsson.[1]

Artificial Intelligence, Machine Learning, Deep Learning, Neural Networks, and Natural Language Processing

Artificial intelligence is the science of building non-human intelligence. Machine learning, deep learning, and natural language processing are subsets of AI. **Machine learning** is a subset of AI that teaches machines to be *smart*. On the other hand, **deep learning** is a subset of machine learning that uses neural networks to solve complex problems. In a nutshell, deep learning is machine learning on an enormous scale, involving millions of training data instances and often multiple layers within the neural network. It is essential that we first know about neural networks.

A **neural network** is a collection of algorithms designed to take in data, then find a solution with the least amount of error. Neural networks form the base of deep learning and are a simple collection of mathematical units organized in layers that work together. Neural networks mimic the structure of a neural circuit in the human brain. A neural circuit is a population of neurons interconnected by synapses to conduct a specific function when activated. Neural networks are made up of layers of neurons or nodes. These nodes are the core processing units of the network. A neural network comprises three layers: input, hidden, and output. Neural networks process data in the input layer; perform most of the computations required by the network, such as recognition of patterns, in the data in the hidden layer; and then predict the final output for a new set of similar data in the output layer. In the past, it was only possible to connect a few layers of nodes due to computing limitations; however, with exponential growth in computational power, it has become possible to build deeper neural networks with more hidden layers that can solve more complex problems and do it faster.

Natural language processing (NLP) is another subset of AI that draws on AI and linguistics to create computer programs that understand human language as it is spoken and written. Examples of NLP include autocomplete and autocorrect on your email or text messages. It also interprets what we mean to say when we talk into our smart speakers or smart devices, such as Alexa, Google Assistant, and Siri. In essence, NLP refers to using computer algorithms to analyze and understand human language as it is spoken or written. This can be done in several ways, including understanding grammar and syntax, identifying keywords and concepts, and even deriving meaning from context.

NLP has a range of potential applications. It can be used for tasks such as sentiment analysis (recognizing positive or negative opinions in text), machine translation, automatic summarization, and information retrieval. Additionally, NLP can help improve communication between humans and computers, for example, by making it easier for people to search for information on the web or by assisting chatbots in understanding customer queries better.

In summary, artificial intelligence, machine learning, and deep learning are interrelated fields. AI is the grand, all-encompassing vision of intelligent machines, and machine learning is the processes and tools taking us there. Machine learning and AI are often used interchangeably. And deep learning is machine learning at the largest scale, with more sophisticated neural networks, exponentially larger datasets, and more robust computing power. However, AI is not restricted to only machine learning and deep learning. AI includes a vast domain of fields, including natural language processing, object detection, computer vision, robotics, and expert systems.

Finally, the word **algorithm** originated in medieval Persia. The term dates back about 900 years. It comes from the name of the Persian mathematical genius, Muhammad ibn Mūsā al'Khwārizmī. The name *Al-Khwarizmi* was Latinized, and it became *alogritmi*, the origin of the word algorithm.[2] But it wasn't until the late 19th century that algorithm came to mean a set of step-by-step rules for solving a problem.

In the early 20th century, Alan Turing theorized how a machine could follow algorithmic instructions to solve complex mathematical problems.[3] This was the birth of the computer age. During World War II, Turing built a machine called the Bombe, which used algorithms to crack the Enigma code, the cipher used by Hitler's army to send messages secretly.

Three significant advances are credited with the recent renaissance of AI:

1. Availability of big data. For computers to achieve learning capabilities, they require lots and lots of data. Large datasets allow AI algorithms to identify patterns, make predictions, and recommend actions. The more, the better.

2. Sophistication and maturity of algorithms. Today, advanced deep learning or machine learning algorithms rely on convolutional or deep neural networks to learn patterns within data and identify possible associations without human intervention.

3. Exponential growth in computation power allows for fast CPU processing. Today, any average game console is more powerful than the computer on Apollo that enabled Neil Armstrong and Buzz Aldrin to take mankind's first steps on the moon.

A Brief History of AI

While Alan Turing is generally considered the founding father of artificial intelligence, it wasn't until 1956 that John McCarthy first coined the official idea and definition of artificial intelligence at the Dartmouth conference. Of course, others had done plenty of research on artificial intelligence before this, but what they were working on was an undefined field before 1956.

In 1950, Alan Turing proposed the Turing test, which is simply a test that determined whether a machine could demonstrate human intelligence. That same year Isaac Asimov proposed the three laws of robotics. In 1951, the first AI-based program was written. In 1955, the first self-learning game-playing program was created. In 1959, the MIT AI Lab was set up. In 1961, the first robot was introduced into General Motors' assembly. 1964 saw the first demo of an AI program that understood natural language. In 1965, the first chatbot, named ELIZA, was invented. In 1974, the first autonomous vehicle was created at Stanford AI Lab. In 1989, Carnegie Mellon made the first autonomous vehicle using a neural network. In 1997, IBM Deep® Blue® beat Garry Kasparov at chess. In 1999, Sony introduced aibo, the first interactive robotic dog. That same year, the MIT AI Lab demonstrated the first emotional AI. In 2004, DARPA introduced the first autonomous vehicle challenge. In 2009, Google started building a self-driving car.

In 2010, Narrative Science's AI demonstrated the ability to write reports. In 2011, IBM Watson beat Jeopardy champions. That same year Siri became mainstream, followed quickly by Google Now and Cortana. In 2015, Elon Musk and others announced a $1 billion donation to launch OpenAI. In 2016, Google DeepMind defeated Go world champion Lee Sedol. Also, in 2016, Stanford University issued the first AI100 report, and UC Berkeley launched the Center for Human-Compatible Artificial Intelligence.

As you can see, AI is not new. Still, the spectacular advances we are making are progressing at an exponential pace, leveraging our ever more powerful computing power, the explosion of digital data, and the speed of communication infrastructure. In some ways, the commercialization era of AI has just begun, and it will profoundly affect our world as we know it as the internet and mobile phones had before, if not more so.

The AI revolution, or the 4th industrial revolution (a term coined in 2016 by Professor Klaus Schwab, the founder of the World Economic Forum), is more important than any other inventions by humankind, including fire and electricity. This spectacular technological invention is superhuman, surpassing our human intelligence. It could be man's last invention. With this in mind, let's begin navigating this complex, exciting field and find out if AI is all it's cracked up to be.

## CHAPTER 3

WHY AI IN MEDICINE?

J ust 30 percent of people believe they're already using AI, while nearly 77 percent are.[4] For good or ill, AI is everywhere. AI recommends the good movies to watch, prevents criminals from using our credit cards, and interprets what we mean when talking to our smart speakers. Today's students are the first generation to grow up with AI.

AI can already do many things that once only humans could do, such as reasoning, adapting, recognizing patterns, and solving complex problems. By 2025, AI will take over more than half of all current work tasks.[5] Employees in every industry will soon work side by side with smart machines to become more efficient and productive, and AI has the power to help us solve some of our biggest problems like climate change, education inequality, and improving global health.

It's nearly impossible to remember when technology did not play a significant role in our lives. But can we rely on computers to detect a cancerous mole? Or can we use a computer algorithm to discern malignancies from benign cellular changes? The use of computerized medical decision-making has been the stuff of sci-fi, but that is rapidly changing, and advances in AI today are transforming our ability to analyze vast quantities of data and predict outcomes in biomedical research, treatment, and healthcare delivery.

A recent physician survey by The Doctors Company, the nation's largest physician-owned medical malpractice insurer, found that 53 percent of physicians are optimistic about the prospects of AI in medicine.[6] A third of US physicians already use AI in their practices, and 66 percent believe AI will lead to faster and more accurate diagnoses.

Many tech aficionados find it tempting to believe that AI and human-centered design technology can be deployed effectively in any situation to serve a need. Still, healthcare is a complex living system and is extremely hard to get right. For AI to make a positive difference, we must carefully consider its ecosystem. What does that healthcare ecosystem look like?

When It Comes to Population Healthcare, What Are Our Unmet Needs?

Our Health Care System Is Wasteful. Healthcare in the US is big business; it is the largest employer in our country, and the per capita spending is staggering. Nearly 19.7 percent of our GDP is spent on healthcare,[7] but when it comes to outcomes, we don't seem to have much to show for it.

When we compare our healthcare system with the other highest-income countries, we discover that we rank first in spending and last in many essential population health outcomes, including obesity, infant mortality, maternal mortality, and life expectancy. To understand why that was the case, McGlynn et al. found that 50 percent of patients were not receiving routine recommended preventative care.[8] At the same time, Ezekiel Emanuel found that our healthcare suffers from **overutilization** of specific medical care compared with other countries.[9] For instance, in the US, costly specialty care, tests, procedures, and prescriptions utilization is 3–5 times higher than in other high-income countries. The cost of exploratory tests and procedures is often just as crippling as the illnesses themselves! And while the total volume of care is not dissimilar to other countries, our cost of care delivery is almost twice as expensive, as reported by Papanicolas et al.[10]

Medical Errors. The US suffers from the same problem of medical errors as the rest of the world. In fact, the US ranks 3rd in **diagnostic errors** compared with other developed countries.[11] Diagnostic errors can lead to patient harm from wrong or delayed testing or treatment. The errors result from several factors, including failing to order the proper tests, misinterpreting test results, not establishing an appropriate differential diagnosis, and missing an abnormal finding. According to The Doctors Company, diagnostic errors are the most significant cause of malpractice claims in the US.[12]

In 2013, Dr. Neill Adhikari found that diagnostic errors have emerged as a global priority in patient safety.[13] Approximately 43 million adverse events occur each year around the globe, which results in 23 million disability-adjusted life years lost and represent a significant source of morbidity and mortality. Many clinicians believe that there is ample reason to think that AI can help address diagnostic errors.

Unmanageable Data. Healthcare data is enormous and complex. It is estimated that medical datasets generate several thousand exabytes of data annually.[14] For comparison, all the internet data available today is approximately hundreds of exabytes. So, yearly medical data is ~ 1000 times more massive than the actual data on our internet.

Can AI help manage the massive amounts of data collected, and can it improve clinical decision-making and diagnosis? Ultimately, can AI affect healthcare and how it is delivered?

Limited Medical Expertise. Clinician shortages are pervasive, especially in low-resource and low-income countries. For instance, there is a severe global shortage of radiologists. Typically, there should be one radiologist to about 12,000 people. However, what's actually seen in developing countries is one radiologist to 200,000 or even 1,000,000 people in the population. There are more radiologists in the Longwood area of Brookline, the geographic domicile of the prestigious institutions Harvard Medical School, the Brigham and Women's Hospital, Boston Children's Hospital, and the Beth Israel Deaconess Medical Center, than in all West Africa! The benefit of AI in healthcare in a region such as West Africa, and other low-resource areas, is that it can help scale up to running some of these complex tasks that would typically require specialized clinicians.

All the above are current problems that AI should fundamentally be able to solve, using machine learning to improve the availability and accuracy of medical care and patient outcomes by scaling and tailoring care to the individual, reducing costs, and reducing medical errors.

When It Comes to Patient Care, What Are Our Unmet Needs? And What Problems Are We Trying to Solve?

So far, we've reviewed where AI could significantly impact healthcare. Now let's look at how AI can make a difference in the lives of individual clinicians.

Human learning is limited by our capacity to remember, access to knowledge sources, and lived experience. Even though there are many brilliant people among us, our limited human brains simply don't have enough memory slots to integrate trends, patterns, and clusters the way computers can. AI can synthesize information from an unlimited number of sources, allowing it to learn at a much faster pace than humans. Machine learning excels in pattern recognition, with machines memorizing those patterns after training on hundreds of thousands, potentially millions, of examples. The history of machine learning has proven that things that are easy for humans can be difficult for machines, and vice versa. Clinicians are not pattern-obsessed freaks, whereas computers are. Conversely, clinicians rely quite a bit on intuition and gut feeling, features machines lack.

There's also a limitation in access to knowledge sources. Despite the advent of the internet and powerful search engines, significant disparities exist in access to good medical information. Another critical challenge is that our learning is primarily derived from lived experiences. We acquire and retain more information from lived experience than any other form of learning. A computer can circumvent all these things. Specific to health-care, just 20 percent of clinicians use evidence to make a diagnosis. The best of us can get the correct diagnosis about 80 percent of the time. No matter what, a clinician will miss one in five diagnoses. With almost 20 percent of the population of the United States visiting an emergency room each year, the population at risk is massive. A large study of ER evaluations of Medicare patients showed that each year more than 10,000 people died within a week of being sent home, despite having no previously diagnosed life-threatening illness.[15] I quote Yuval Noah Harari, who wrote the book *Homo Deus,* "Alas, not even the most diligent doctor can remember all my previous ailments and checkups."[16] Similarly, no clinician can be familiar with every illness and drug or read every new article published in every medical journal. Additionally, the clinician is sometimes tired, hungry, or perhaps even sick, affecting their judgment. No wonder clinicians sometimes err in their diagnosis or recommend a less than optimal treatment.

AI algorithms don't suffer from recency or other cognitive biases. That's not to say that an algorithm cannot be biased—but that is not a cognitive bias. Misdiagnoses and errors in judgment often result from cognitive biases and distortions. Our modest minds always seek one simple, straightforward, unifying diagnosis, or whatever instantly pops into our minds based on past experiences or the last patient we saw: the recency bias. In his masterful book *Deep Medicine,*[17] Dr. Eric Topol states, "There are about 10,000 human diseases, and there's not a doctor who could recall any significant fraction of them. If doctors can't remember a possible diagnosis when making up a differential, then they will diagnose according to the possibilities that are mentally available to them, and an error can result. This is called the availability bias."

"A second bias results from the fact that doctors deal with patients one at a time. In 1990, a study in the *New England Journal of Medicine* showed how individual patients, especially patients that a doctor has recently seen, can shape medical judgment simply because each doctor only sees a relatively small number of patients. Their personal experience as doctors can override hard data derived from much larger samples of people say about the likelihood that a patient has some rare disease simply because an earlier patient with similar symptoms had that rare disease," remarked Dr. Topol.[18]

Of course, it follows that over two million medication errors are made every year.[19] To compound the problem further, the medical literature—which is already quite exhaustive—doubles every five years; hence, our fund of scientific knowledge doubles. You can see how difficult it would be to keep up to date with all the clinical knowledge.

Furthermore, most of us (80 percent) spend less than five hours per month reading medical literature.[20] It is estimated that more than two million research papers are published yearly. In PubMed, there are more than 27 million research papers.[21] Even if one could read five papers in their field of interest per week, it's still impossible to stay abreast of everything published in a lifetime. Meanwhile, a staggering number of new studies are cranked out every day. To keep up with all the published medical research, a clinician must read 5000 journal articles daily. On the other hand, IBM's AI program, Watson, can process a million pages in seconds. It's inconceivable for a clinician (or any human being) to keep current with the medical literature, live everyday life, have a family, exercise, and perform other activities of daily living.

So, what potential benefits can be derived from AI-augmented knowledge in medicine? By knowing more data and getting our arms around more information, we can make better clinical decisions and more accurate diagnoses. This is particularly pertinent in radiology, dermatology, and pathology, clinical fields, which tend to be more image oriented. We may be able to keep up to date with the information we need from medical journals and textbooks without succumbing to burnout from exhaustion and emotional instability, the hallmarks of moral injury.

Making better decisions and exhibiting better judgment may also catapult a fresh clinician into an experienced one because, as I mentioned earlier, experience in clinical medicine is a lived one. Ostensibly through AI, the less experienced can hone their skills faster and become more proficient.

AI doesn't get emotional, need a vacation, get overworked, feel overwhelmed, or get sick (although it can glitch or stop working altogether)! It's unwavering, objective, and unaffected by our common limitations of fatigue, sleep deprivation, bad days, or distraction. And, of course, AI technology is available 24/7. The benefits of AI in medicine should precisely translate to early detection and a better understanding of disease progression, perhaps enabling us to optimize and personalize treatment and, in many cases, uncover novel treatments that were not readily obvious, i.e., sharpen our clinical acumen. These benefits are particularly valuable in low-resource settings where socioeconomic inequity and healthcare disparity are more pronounced because of general shortages of physicians and providers.

The aha moment in healthcare—what put AI on the map—was when IBM Watson, the cousin of IBM® Deep Blue®—which went to medical school—was pitted against the elite, world-renowned oncologists from the University of North Carolina. The competition was whether the AI algorithm could accurately predict the correct treatment for cancer diagnoses. Watson was tested on 1,000 cancer diagnoses made by human experts. In 99 percent of the cancer diagnoses, Watson recommended the same treatment as the oncologists. In 30 percent of the cases, Watson also found a treatment option that human doctors had missed. Some treatments were based on research papers the doctors had not read, as more than 160,000 cancer research papers are published annually. In addition, Watson uncovered other novel treatment options that had surfaced in new clinical trials that the oncologists had not yet seen announced on the web.[22] Obviously, it's impractical, if not impossible, for an oncologist, even the most dedicated, to keep abreast of all that colossal literature. Not only did Watson get the treatment right, but it suggested treatment protocols that weren't apparent to these elite oncologists!

While this wasn't "game over" for human medicine, it got our attention. The explosion of new ideas and applications of AI in medicine followed. Inevitably, AI in medicine has since experienced exponential growth in academic institutions. Of course, academic centers are not the only groups pursuing technology. The private sector is entirely on board, backed by major private equity and venture capital funding, with a keen interest in all fields of healthcare, such as robot-assisted surgery, virtual nursing assistance, administrative workflow assistance, cyber security and fraud detection, dosage error reduction, clinical trials, medical diagnosis, and automated image diagnosis, to name a few. There is also an extensive collaboration between academia and the private sector. For instance, Google DeepMind Health, in collaboration with Stanford, UCSF, and the University of Chicago, has developed machine learning models which could accurately predict multiple medical events using reams of electronic health records data. The model proved that it could accurately predict numerous medical events like unexpected readmissions or length of stay. This means that doctors can now make assessments and generate new hypotheses from the information in the electronic health records, a significant pain point clinicians face daily. We know that six hours of an average clinician's 11-hour workday can be spent on the chart. Fortunately, we are at a point where AI can offload those six hours and give the time back to the clinician.

In conclusion, potential benefits of AI in medicine include aid with medical diagnosis, integration, and improvement of workflow, enhanced image scanning and segmentation, supported decision making, and disease risk prediction. AI holds so much promise, yet it is not without challenges; many people are unsure of its effectiveness and reliability. Understandably, we must consider the future role of clinicians and what unforeseen impact AI will have on our job security. Forty percent of jobs in the world will be displaced by technology.[23] Should we be worried about our jobs?

In the ensuing chapters, I will focus on the AI applications that could augment or change clinical practice and discuss AI's pros, cons, biases, and pitfalls. Invariably, these benefits must outweigh the risks of wide AI adoption in medicine. I will explore examples of some of the significant and most impactful AI innovations in medicine that are already in progress and that are expected to manifest even more meaningfully in the next few years.

## CHAPTER 4

THE DREADED ELECTRONIC HEALTH RECORD

The Problems

Who doesn't think that the electronic health record (EHR) should be reformed? I do! This is undoubtedly the most excruciating pain point the clinician faces daily. Up to six hours of an eleven-hour workday can be spent agonizingly reviewing charts. That's more than 50 percent of our clinical time! For every hour we spend with the patient, we spend another two hours on the EHR, not to mention another hour at night with our inbox.

These bureaucratic tasks involved in managing health IT and EHR systems are, in fact, among the most cited causes of clinician burnout. More than half of the burnout cases in medicine are attributable to the EHR. In 2017, Robertson et al. conducted 600 anonymous surveys of residents and faculty in 19 primary care programs about burnout and satisfaction with work-life balance. The results were startling! Respondents who spent more than six hours weekly after office hours in EHR work were three times more likely to report burnout and four times more likely to attribute burnout to the EHR.[24]

Is it surprising then that the prevalence of clinician burnout correlates with the widespread use of the EHR? In a national survey in 2008, only 13 percent of physicians reported having a basic EHR system. By the end of 2012, 72 percent of physicians had adopted some EHR system, and 40 percent of physicians reported having capabilities that met the criteria for a basic system.[25]

Clinician burnout is a new illness rampant in this community of highly educated and trained individuals. Among those affected, it causes impaired professionalism, higher rates of depression, and even suicidal ideation and suicidality. The prevalence in clinicians is 54 percent; however, in some specialties, such as primary care and emergency medicine, more than 60 percent are affected. Approximately 500,000 clinicians are affected, a prevalence comparable to lung cancer. Dr. Phillip Kroth, director of Biomedical Informatics Research at UNM, remarked, "We are losing the equivalent of seven graduating classes of physicians yearly to burnout and, as they leave the profession, they point their finger at the time now required for them to document their work and how it has led to the loss of quality time spent with patients and families."[26]

Healthcare organizations have seen real clinical and financial benefits with the widespread adoption of the EHR. In addition to giving clinicians access to patients' information with just a few clicks, data tools within the EHR promote appropriate care decisions and reduce medical errors. However, EHR usability issues make working in the system remarkably time consuming and frustrating.

I'm sure many of you are familiar with the satirical cartoons depicting a modern clinician in a white coat with a stethoscope around their neck, not sitting across from a patient but staring instead at a glowing monitor and clicking away on a keyboard.

According to Dr. Topol in *Deep Medicine*, the median clinic visit length in the US is 13 minutes for a new patient and 7 minutes for an established one.[27] Sadly, 90 percent of the clinical encounter is spent on digesting data, leaving the remaining one to two minutes for direct eye contact with the patient. No wonder patients are frustrated! Again, Dr. Topol wrote, "Both patients and doctors believe that doctors are rushed. Recently, for example, the Medical Center at the University of Alabama at Birmingham asked patients what two words best describe its doctors. The partial response is telling. Rude, hurried, brief, rushed. Busy. Unconcerned. Poor. Condescending."

A 2019 study published in the *Annals of Internal Medicine* unsurprisingly confirmed what clinicians have long believed: Physicians spend much more time entering data than talking directly with patients.[28] The study was conducted by researchers from Dartmouth-Hitchcock health system, the American Medical Association (AMA), Sharp End Advisory, and the Australian Institute of Health Innovation (AIHI), and it cut across the disciplines of medicine. In four states, they observed 57 US providers who practiced cardiology, family medicine, orthopedics, or internal medicine. They followed the physicians for 430 work hours, and 21 providers kept journals to log any after-hours work. They reported that physicians spent less than a third of the clinic day on direct clinical face time with patients, whereas 50 percent of their time was spent on EHRs and other desk work. When in the examination room with patients, physicians spent 52.9 percent of their time directly talking with patients and 37 percent on EHR and other desk work, including reviewing test results, logging information, and writing medication orders. This diminishes the quality time you spend with your patient when the whole idea is to be present, develop rapport with the patient, and be patient-centered; the primary reason many of us became clinicians and the essence of the medical profession. This also means that without the excessive administrative and bureaucratic tasks, clinicians could see more patients, and patients would not have to wait as long to be seen. This increases efficiency and productivity; both urgently needed solutions. The EHR seems to satisfy government regulations and maximization of reimbursement from billing rather than the needs of providers and patients. And despite spending half of the workday on EHR, physicians spend two hours of their personal time every night catching up on data entry work. These results are depressing, perhaps even incriminating, as they could be directly linked to rising physician burnout rates when an estimated 300 to 400 doctors die by suicide each year in the US.[29]

Let's specifically examine some of the disadvantages of the EHR. In addition to detracting from a proper encounter with our patients, the EHR is often fragmented and incomplete. It takes excessive time to train a provider to use it. It's frequently not completely digitized; usually, there are accompanying scanned or faxed notes. It's often clunky; it can be slow, freeze, or stop working altogether. And most important, the majority of the EHR notes are cloned. According to a *JAMA Internal Medicine* paper published in 2017, more than 80 percent of the notes in the EHR were imported or copied from elsewhere.[30] This cloning of notes increases the risk of including outdated, inaccurate, or unnecessary information, which can undermine the utility of notes and lead to a clinical error.

The Solutions

Imagine if you can devote the time it takes to deal with administrative tasks and technology (e.g., inputting information, searching for faxes, labs, diagnostic test results, etc.) to the patients instead. That would be a massive step towards becoming a better clinician! Giving us back that valuable time will free us to dedicate ourselves to our patients. Imagine if a clinician could get all the information needed about a patient in two minutes and then spend the next eleven minutes of the office visit talking with the patient instead of the other way around, our current status quo.

The EHR is the avenue requiring the most disruption and overhaul; the patient encounter is the area of greatest need for a smart EHR that can use speech recognition and natural language processing to relieve the clinical documentation burden. Imagine if you can walk into an exam room, make full eye contact, and converse with your patient. Complete a physical exam and discuss treatment options. All relevant clinical information has been captured and documented by the time you are ready to leave the room. The clinical orders have been placed, the note has been completed, and charges have been generated.

This dream of a simpler, efficient, and more productive interaction with our patients is fast becoming a reality. It may become actionable sooner than we think. Technology to be fitted into the exam room would include microphones, videos, and sensors to observe our interactions with the patient. Think of an Alexa-like device in the room that listens to and records everything. The encounter can be transcribed and correlated with non-verbal sensor data, creating a compelling, concise summary of the visit. Next, this smart EHR will assist with medical decision-making.

As providers and patients interact in real-time, the smart AI algorithm can generate a differential diagnosis based on the newly acquired data from the conversation and sensor data and display it on the in-room monitor. AI can then comb through the literature in real time—all the thousands, millions of clinical papers in existence—and extract all the best practices and pathways that can be matched to your patient.

What if the computer was smart enough to listen in when I'm talking to the patient, use natural language processing to record the conversation, and transcribe the medical note (the clerical task) while simultaneously synthesizing this information in the background alerting me in real time? "I heard this patient coughing. The pattern of cough suggests asthma. She works in a factory manufacturing paint and varnishes; therefore, she's at risk for occupational asthma. I suspect exposure to chlorine or ammonia, or diesel exhaust fumes. I suggest you ask her if she's short of breath and whether the factory uses diesel or these other chemicals?"

This would be a truly smart EHR, guiding me to improve my interview and information acquisition, alerting me to the likely diagnosis, and recommending the best treatment. I can also focus on the patient rather than be distracted by a keyboard and a screen.

Furthermore, the algorithm may assist with identifying potential gaps in care, including necessary treatments and care pathways to better manage the patient's chronic conditions and lessen our tendency to focus on only the urgent problem or the "tyranny of the acute." Inevitably, this diagnosis and management assistance or augmentation should lead to better patient care and treatment outcomes, perhaps even predict whether this patient will develop other diseases, such as diabetes or kidney failure, depression, or be a victim of domestic abuse within the next 12 months. This will surely make us work *smarter.*

AI Applications to Provide EHR Solutions

Reduce Administrative Burden of Clinical Documentation. By developing AI algorithms to study the clinical workflow and facilitate the clinical visit capturing process using automatic speech recognition, the goal is to reduce that administrative burden and give the gift of time back to clinicians so they can focus on the patient.

The American Academy of Family Physicians (AAFP) has launched a series of Innovation Labs to identify and demonstrate tech solutions essential to optimizing the family medicine experience.[31] The Innovation Lab partnered with Suki Digital Assistant, which was already in use by some family physicians, who found it easily implementable and affordable. Their lab proved that using an AI assistant can significantly reduce the enormous documentation burden and family physician burnout.

Of the 132 physicians and clinicians studied, 102 completed the trial, and 61 participants fully adopted the solution as paying customers after the lab, a 60 percent adoption rate. The participants reported a 72 percent reduction in their median documentation time per note and 76 percent during after-hours, which was called a "breakthrough" by some clinicians. This resulted in a calculated time savings of 3.3 hours per week per clinician. The following are quotes from some family physicians who participated in the trial:

> *"Now, I finish up about 30 minutes after clinic is done and after those 30 minutes, I'm not typically taking anything home."*
>
> *"Just the ability to give you back control of your time. So, at lunch, if I felt like I was getting behind and I needed to go to the next room before completing documentation, I could do it at lunchtime. And I could do it before I need to leave to go home."*

Other companies in this field include Nuance, 3M™ M*Modal, iScribe, Amazon Transcribe Medical, Robin Healthcare, and the tech giants Microsoft, Apple, and Google.

Automated Extraction of Patient Information. Patient data must be easily accessible to providers for faster diagnosis and decision-making. Moreover, it should be straightforward to read for clinicians to interpret the data accurately. But sorting through substantial amounts of EHR data and picking the bits that apply to a patient's condition is tedious, impractical, and nearly impossible.

AI-enabled EHR systems can allow clinicians to rapidly access, extract, and electronically export patient data with minimal error. For instance, One Medical enables data extraction from clinical documents using athenahealth's AI-enabled cloud-based EHR. Flatiron Health's AI can review provider notes and extract structured data. Additionally, Amazon Web Services recently launched a cloud-based service called Amazon Comprehend Medical that can retrieve and index data from clinical notes. Other companies in this area include Concord Technologies, Linguamatics, Innodata Inc., and Intellidact AI.

Enhanced Clinical Decision-Making. The AAFP is collaborating with Navina Lab; an AI-driven point-of-care platform that facilitates real-time access and analysis of patient data to optimize diagnosis and ICD coding processes for proper payment. Other companies in this area include Google, Change Healthcare, AllScripts, Jvion , and Epic Systems' AI solutions.

CMS Artificial Intelligence Health Outcomes Challenge. The Centers for Medicare & Medicaid Services (CMS) challenge engages innovators from all sectors—not just healthcare—to harness AI solutions that can predict health outcomes for potential adoption and use in the CMS Innovation Center's payment and service delivery models.

The potential for increased AI usage in medicine is not just in reducing manual tasks and freeing up physicians' time, increasing efficiency and productivity; it also presents the opportunity for us to move towards more precision medicine. As summarized by Bertalan Meskó, MD, Ph.D. in an article for LinkedIn, "Artificial narrow intelligence (ANI) will most likely help healthcare move from traditional, 'one-size-fits-all' medical solutions towards targeted treatments, personalized therapies, and uniquely composed drugs."[32]

For many years and by necessity, general practice in medicine has been to gather data and generalize. As Meskó puts it, treatment is often based on the needs of the statistically average person. With the advent of precision medicine, that paradigm is quickly changing. Now we are in an age where reams of data that reflect differences in patients' genes, environments, and lifestyles can be collected and rapidly analyzed. Developing individualized treatments based on this specific knowledge is becoming more feasible. Statistics will no longer dictate your health fate; individuals now hold power over proactive decision-making processes through the data gathered about themselves. In other words: YOU are your own best doctor! Demonstrating this shift, last year, Google released an open-source version of DeepVariant, an AI tool for precision medicine. Rivals IBM and

Microsoft are also moving into the healthcare IT space, with speculation that Apple and Amazon will soon do the same.

Final Thoughts

Physicians, nurses, and other clinicians often spend more time on administrative tasks, such as entering data into EHRs. This is contributing to high levels of burnout among these professionals. A recent study at the University of Colorado found that taking the computer out of the exam room and supporting doctors with human medical assistants led to a striking reduction in physician burnout, from 53 percent to 13 percent.[33]

Projecting these findings to other healthcare settings, it is clear that freeing up clinicians' time will significantly improve patient care. For example, if 25 percent more time can be released for nurses across different specialties, this would result in an estimated 1.5 million more hours available for direct patient care each year. Similarly, if 25 percent more time can be cleared for clinicians across different specialties, this would result in an estimated 10 million more hours available for direct patient care each year.

This extra time will improve patients' outcomes and reduce costs by lessening the need for expensive medical interventions. Given all these benefits, freeing clinicians' time should be a top priority for healthcare organizations worldwide.

## CHAPTER 5

MISDIAGNOSIS

A 59-year-old man was found by his wife to be lethargic after a nap. The husband had recently had a cold but felt he was "over it." He had also returned from a business trip the previous night.

By the time he got to the ER, he was found to have weakness and complained of hoarseness and blurry vision. He intimated to the ER doc that he had a medication change one week ago and was on an opioid medication for long-standing back pain. The ER doc decided to order a head CT scan, even though she had a low index of suspicion for a stroke, and it was negative for any acute findings. Strokes can be challenging to diagnose, and it's essential to rule them out completely. The decision to order a CT scan was the right call. The patient was then discharged with a diagnosis of upper respiratory infection and advised to discontinue his opioid medication.

At home, the patient continued to have intermittent lethargy and hypersomnia, alternating with agitation and delirium. Eventually, he became unresponsive. His wife called 9-1-1, and he was again rushed to the hospital ER. An urgent non-contrast CT was negative, followed by CT angiography, which confirmed basilar artery occlusion, one of the worst and often fatal complications of a posterior stroke. Misdiagnosis, delay in diagnosis, and failure to recognize a complication were the trifecta that led to this fateful outcome, this young patient's untimely death.

A posterior circulation stroke is a rare stroke affecting the back part of the brain. This type of stroke can cause balance, movement, and vision problems. An index of suspicion for posterior circulation stroke (PCS) would have potentially saved this patient's life. An urgent diffusion magnetic resonance imaging (MRI) or CT angiogram (not non-contrast CT) would have shown basilar artery occlusion. And suppose the patient was a candidate for thrombolysis therapy, intravenous tissue-type plasminogen activator (tPA), or acute endovascular therapy (intra-arterial clot removal or lysis, usually employed within 4.5 hours of symptom onset to prevent the high likelihood of death or severe disability which a basilar artery stroke can cause). In that case, that may just have saved his life.

This unfortunate example highlights and encapsulates the problem with misdiagnosing something as apparent as a stroke. Ischemic strokes comprise 87 percent of all strokes, and approximately 20 percent of ischemic strokes are posterior strokes, three times more likely to be misdiagnosed.[34] Typical symptoms are the 5 Ds of posterior stroke: dizziness, diplopia, dysarthria, dysphagia, and dystaxia.[35]

Our patient had three of the Ds: blurry vision (diplopia), hoarseness (dysarthria), and weakness (dizziness). However, PCS is a vexing entity for clinicians because of the myriad of ways it can present, ranging from the obvious to the mundane. It is probably more common than generally appreciated. For example, vertigo is a frequent symptom of PCS but is non-specific, meaning it doesn't immediately give away the diagnosis.

Unfortunately, neither the case nor the setting is unique. As many as 165,000 strokes yearly may be misdiagnosed in US emergency rooms. In this high turnover place, a clinician must rapidly determine whether to discharge or admit the patient. A wrong diagnosis could be a matter of life and death. The scope of this problem is enormous; 20 percent of the US population visits emergency rooms each year.[36] Obermeyer et al. published a study in 2017 that showed that every year, 10,000 Medicare beneficiaries die within seven days after discharge from emergency rooms, despite no documented suspicion of life-threatening illnesses.[37] The mean age at death of these patients was 69. As we will see in the following example, misdiagnosis is not exclusively the purview of the emergency room.

Sarah was considered a medical mystery. It began when she was 18. She had several bouts of abdominal pain and fevers. Multiple visits to the hospital, countless tests, and even surgeries did not disclose a definitive diagnosis. It happened again and again and again for the next three years. The doctors were at a loss for what could be wrong with her. She had undergone every test imaginable to no avail. No one could tell her what was wrong with her body. Finally, after years of suffering, an infectious disease specialist at Johns Hopkins Hospital diagnosed Sarah with Fitz-Hugh–Curtis syndrome (FHC), a rare pelvic inflammatory disease (PID) complication. This infection starts in the vagina or cervix and spreads to the liver. FHC leads to inflammation of the liver and scarring around the gallbladder. The symptoms mimic other diseases, so it often goes undiagnosed for years. This doctor made the correct diagnosis because he recognized a pattern in her symptoms; he had seen it before.

"It's clear from some of the earliest research that's been done on the diagnosis that the person or doctor most likely to get the right answer is the person or doctor who has seen something before," remarked Dr. Lisa Sanders, a Yale internist. The latter writes the famous and brilliant Diagnosis column for *New York Times Magazine*. Her column-inspired

House MD, a once-popular TV show, for which she also served as a consultant. Dr. Sanders and the New York Times created Diagnosis, a Netflix documentary series on the diagnosis process.

In this series, baffling and elusive illnesses are diagnosed not solely by medical experts but by crowdsourcing: using audiences worldwide to search for anybody who might recognize and identify a patient's condition. In her column and series, Dr. Sanders spotlights people with undiagnosed illnesses. The stories go up on the internet and open the door for medical professionals, amateur medical detectives, and anyone else to offer their two cents. A GoFundMe for information instead of money, if you will.

Other crowdsourcing diagnostic platforms exist. For instance, the organization CrowdMed crowdsources diagnoses using a network of "medical detectives," including physicians, healthcare practitioners, and other people, some of whom aren't medically trained. A review of CrowdMed's efficacy in 2016 noted that, while CrowdMed has cracked various cases, a large proportion of the medical detectives don't have medical degrees, and their ability to give diagnoses could be an issue of legal concern.[38]

While benevolent, these crowdsourcing platforms represent a desperate and deplorable state of affairs when we must rely on other medical professionals, students, and some people without medical training to crack a tricky diagnosis. They highlight the fragmentation of our health system and the non-democratized access to knowledge and expertise, even in the wealthiest country in the world.

Fortunately, we have Medscape Consult, a doctors-only consulting platform connecting physicians worldwide to communicate about cases. A review of the platform in 2018 found that 37,000 physicians used it from every continent.[39] Many minds and perspectives can be far better than one.

The Problems

Sarah's case represents just one of 7000 known rare diseases. More are found every year. Some 30 million Americans have these rare diseases.[40] And like Sarah, many have trouble finding out what's making them sick. The average time to diagnosis is six years. Why does it take so long? Why do doctors have trouble identifying diseases affecting 1 in 10 Americans? Honestly, we're not just missing the rare ones. I don't intend to go too deep into the nitty-gritty of how clinicians diagnose but would recommend Dr. Eric Topol's exceptional book, *Deep Medicine*.[41]

When a patient goes to their doctor, it's usually with what they consider a simple question: What's the diagnosis? Well, how do we reach a diagnosis? We know that common presentations tend to repeat. This is the basis of Bayes' theorem, a tool of statistical inference which relies on prior occurrences.[42] Most of us see a few thousand patients in our lifetime. That seems like a vast number, but it is hardly an extensive database. The older and more experienced clinicians are inevitably better diagnosticians because they have seen tens of thousands of patients.

"And before I started medical school, I thought the answer to that question was simple, like the multiplication table 4 x 6 is always 24, so fever and a rash would always be the same predictable entity. But of course, that's not the case. Not even close. A fever and a rash could have dozens of causes, including viral infections like measles or chickenpox. It could indicate a severe allergic reaction. It could be the first sign of hidden cancer. You see, diagnosis, it's not math, it's Sherlock Holmes," affirms Dr. Sanders.[43]

We make at least 12 million misdiagnoses every year. 90,000 people die in the hospital annually because of missed or wrong diagnoses. That exceeds the number of people that were killed at the peak of the opioid epidemic.[44] The National Academy of Medicine published a report on diagnostic error in 2015 that brings it closer to home.[45] Their account opens with the line that most of us will be subject to at least one diagnostic error in our lifetime, and some of these errors will have tragic consequences.

Even the cleverest of clinicians will get it wrong one in five times, and the second opinion diagnosis agrees with the referral physician's diagnosis in only 12 percent of patients.[46]

What constitutes a misdiagnosis?

- Wrong diagnosis
- Failing to order the proper test
- Misinterpretation of the test
- Missed abnormal result
- Delayed diagnosis

Let's look at an average clinician. New diagnostic tests, treatments, and guidelines will regularly appear for the hundreds of different common conditions that they see. Suppose they are a cancer specialist, for example. In that case, new subsegments of disease are discovered by mutational or phenotypic analysis, new drugs or cell therapies are emerging from laboratories, and patients appear with unusual combinations of comorbidities or pathologies these specialists have never seen before but suspect others have.

An average clinician usually sees 20,000 patients during their career. Interestingly, there is no formal system to give clinicians feedback about whether their diagnoses were correct. For example, suppose we miss a diagnosis, and a patient develops cancer three years later. In that case, no formal system provides a feedback loop to help us learn from our mistakes and improve our future diagnostic accuracy. It takes many decades for each clinician to accumulate first-hand experience, which is still limited, even for the clinician who regularly consumes a heavy volume of literature and might see tens of thousands of patients throughout a career. This experience is negligible compared with what could be collected by AI, which can ingest data from all 700,000 physicians and nearly 500,000 nurse practitioners and physician assistants currently practicing in the United States and the several million worldwide. Imagine harnessing the de-identified data of millions, possibly billions, of patients to assist clinicians with making a diagnosis; every past medical decision could help inform every future medical decision.

The task of staying current is now beyond the capability of any clinician; it's almost superhuman, one may say. The average clinician usually has five or fewer differential diagnoses for every patient presentation. This is out of nearly 10,000 human diseases. Only with AI augmentation can it be humanly possible to incorporate all these differential diagnoses on one's list.

While many biases potentially affect our judgment and cause diagnostic errors, the following three appear to be the most common.

The first is the **availability bias**. A clinician usually diagnoses based on the mental possibilities available to them. Even for those with an extensive fund of medical knowledge, 10,000 human disease possibilities are overwhelming. A large study of 583 doctor-reported cases of diagnostic errors concluded that the biggest problem in diagnostic failure was not considering the diagnosis in the first place.[47] This is partly an example of the availability bias.

The second is the **recency bias**. Given that most clinicians only see a relatively small number of patients, a recent patient with an unusual diagnosis usually has an outsized influence or bias on their medical judgment; we continue to think about that diagnosis with subsequent patients.

The third, and most prevalent bias among physicians, is **overconfidence**. A study showed that clinicians who were 'completely certain' of the diagnosis antemortem were wrong 40 percent of the time at autopsy.

An outgrowth of overconfidence is the last, which is the **confirmation bias**. This can be described as the inclination to make decisions by considering only the information that is consistent with one's existing beliefs. A clinician will unintentionally reject all the inconsistent information with a particular diagnosis.

Failure to recognize these cognitive biases and the lack of feedback on our diagnostic performance leads us to develop lifelong mistakes, and worse, we are not even aware they exist!

As we saw in Chapter 3, the healthcare system is wasteful. Reducing this waste will require addressing multiple sources of unnecessary spending, one of which is inappropriate clinical decision-making. Failure to diagnose or delay in diagnosis are the most cited reasons for malpractice litigation in the United States, which in 2017 accounted for 31 percent of lawsuits.[48]

Assimilating all available information is challenging even with unlimited time and resources. Dr. Kohane, Professor of Bioinformatics at Harvard Medical School and leader in machine learning, argues that, despite the critical importance of historical data in medical decision-making and the growing amount of longitudinal data available in EHR systems, clinicians typically do not have the time or the resources to review this information during a clinical visit thoroughly.[49] *Tyranny of the urgent* was coined to describe that brief patient-doctor visit that allows time enough to deal only with acute situations rather than optimize long-term care.[50] As a result, much of the electronic health information might not be appropriately interpreted, utilized, or accessed, leading to potentially missed diagnoses of specific clinical conditions.

Kohane concludes that we must obey our limitations as human beings who are error-prone and who must ultimately rely on process automation. "The best way is to change medical education. To make doctors think of medicine as a data processing endeavor," Kohane said. If it makes you, the clinician, feel better, the blame for diagnostic errors can't be entirely laid at our doorstep. It is not just an individual-level failure but also a failure at the population level. The healthcare system is frequently blind and miscues data that's staring us in the face.

Dr. Kohane told a story of the Malaysian airliner that disappeared in March 2014 and how the entire world was activated to figure out where it had gone and what had happened. Meanwhile, two of the top hospitals in Boston experienced a peak in heart attacks. As it happened, an 18 percent increase over baseline was seen in heart attacks. Nearly 1000 planeloads of patients with heart attacks. And guess what? No one noticed. It's only when they analyzed the electronic health record of the data that we first became aware of it. "So, it's like 1000 Malaysian 747s disappeared without a trace before we noticed this," said Kohane. The cause was eventually determined to be Vioxx, a COX-2 inhibitor, anti-inflammatory pain medication with severe cardiotoxicity. Vioxx was then quickly black-boxed and then shut down by the FDA.

He continued, "I'd get a standing ovation maybe if I told you that we had caused a 5 percent decrease in heart attacks. Instead, we caused an 18 percent increase in heart attacks, and we didn't even know it. And it was notable. Interestingly, Kaiser Permanente took it off their formulary early on when they saw early papers suggesting that there was cardiotoxicity. However, that information had not reached even two of the world's most prominent hospitals. That's our healthcare system. And guess what? This is still happening now, today. We're not paying attention... We're missing huge signals if we could only bother to be creative, which are very plain to see once you bother looking on the record."

Clinicians are often inundated with data that is often contradictory and chaotic. And while they may have years of schooling and experience, this does not mean they can deal with every situation. Again, the task of staying current is now beyond the capability of any clinician. Medicine generates vast data that exceeds our capacity to process and use it effectively and efficiently.

Reis et al. aggregated all the ICD 9 discharge codes across Massachusetts.[51] The researchers used EHR data from 500,000 Massachusetts patients. They developed an AI model to predict a patient's risk of receiving a future abuse diagnosis based on the patient's longitudinal diagnostic record. The model could predict the diagnosis of domestic abuse two years, on average, in advance of the confirmation. This prediction can help caregivers identify individuals who fall into either of two categories: those who may be currently experiencing abuse but have yet to be diagnosed and those who are not yet experiencing abuse but are at a high risk of being abused in the future.

Yuval Barak-Corren used longitudinal EHR data to predict patients' future risk of suicidal behavior.[52] The model achieved 33 percent sensitivity, 95 percent specificity, and early (3–4 years in advance on average) prediction of patients' future suicidal behavior. A similar predictive model was validated in psychiatry. The researchers concluded that this modeling approach could serve as an early warning system to help clinicians identify high-risk patients for further screening. By analyzing the full phenotypic breadth of the EHR, computerized risk screening approaches may enhance prediction beyond what is possible for the individual clinician.

We are not even good at statistics! A group of Harvard and Boston University medical school students, residents, and attendings were asked, "If a test to detect a disease whose prevalence is 1/1000 has a false positive rate of 5 percent, what is the chance that a person found to have a positive result actually has the disease, assuming you know nothing about the person's symptoms or signs?" The most common answer was 95 percent.[53] The correct answer is 2 percent. Let me illustrate this arithmetic. For every true positive in, say, 1000 individuals, there are 5 percent false positives or 50 people. Including the true positives that we have, we have 51 positives. So, it's a 1/51 chance of a true positive. Ninety-five percent got this wrong. And by the way, this same study was published 30 years prior in the *New England Journal of Medicine*, and the Harvard doctors were no better then.[54] One could conclude that most clinicians can't calculate basic statistics, which is unlikely to change. "What if we did this across thousands of expensive somatic genomic sequencing tests? Imagine how this would make the false positive disasters of mammography and prostate-specific antigen look like chump change, with patients subjected to more unnecessary and expensive tests, procedures, and possibly even surgeries for false positives," concluded Kohane.

A 2022 study by Zirui Song at Harvard Medical School looked at variability in physician decision-making.[55] The researchers studied situations where clear-cut guidelines have been in place for years. The study found that the physicians who made the most clinically appropriate decisions were five to ten times more likely to have used evidence-based care than their peers whose decisions tended to be the least appropriate. In other words, evidence-based clinical decisions trump those that are non-evidence-based!

To make matters worse, even clinicians who adhere to evidence-based medicine are often challenged. Some clinical situations are complex, requiring physicians to make clinical decisions without the benefit of guidelines or evidence-based care standards and choose from options that involve substantial uncertainty for patient outcomes.

The Solutions

The advent of advanced analytic methodologies for large, complex datasets and the development of machine learning techniques—where computers process enormous amounts of data to learn from examples rather than be preprogrammed with rules based on human inputs—will likely lead to the development of progressively more powerful and sophisticated clinical decision support systems. AI systems are increasingly used in a diagnostic role within clinical settings. Engineers have developed AI machines that analyze previous patient records, primarily their symptoms and subsequent diagnoses, and then use that information to diagnose new patients. These machines often learn as they encounter further patient information, increasing diagnostic accuracy. In essence, the machines mimic the way a clinician would process relevant medical information and then come to a diagnosis. AI can even mine medical records, social media, physical findings, labs, imaging, and genomic data to predict probabilities and generate the best insights.

At Guangzhou Women and Children's Medical Center in China, researchers developed an AI-based system to test the accuracy of machine learning in diagnosing common pediatric conditions.[56] Researchers used existing patient records to train the system. To compare the accuracy of the AI system with actual physicians, they inputted different patient records into the system and allowed the system to predict a diagnosis. Then they compared the system's diagnosis with the real physician's diagnosis. In total, over one million existing pediatric records were used to train and validate the system's accuracy. The system had a precision comparable to that of experienced pediatricians, especially in common conditions like acute respiratory infections, bronchitis, and tonsillitis.

As we saw from the domestic abuse study,[57] potential next steps towards developing an early warning system for clinicians would include automation of the intelligent history tool, as well as refinement and testing of the numerical and visual presentations of the human interface.

The general model has far-reaching potential implications for automated screening of other clinical conditions where longitudinal historical information can be used to predict the patient's clinical risk. The approach would work as follows: A patient's longitudinal medical history accumulates over time inside an EHR system. Whenever new information is recorded for the patient, the intelligent histories model re-analyzes the data gathered to estimate the patient's risk of receiving a future diagnosis of clinical condition x. The provider is notified if the patient is at substantial risk for x. The provider uses the visualization to quickly review the patient's past diagnoses and identify critical long-term trends in the patient's history. The risk estimate, together with the high-level view of the patient's diagnostic history, enables the clinician to make a better-informed decision about further patient screening. In this way, the intelligent histories model could improve screening by helping clinicians identify high-risk patients who might otherwise be missed.

Clinicians and the health systems in which they work can become members of an extended 'clinical knowledge network,' sharing and receiving the insights that transcend any practice or geographical area. Overall, the effect will democratize access to clinical knowledge, both to current best practices and specific learnings from comparable individual cases in rare and complex conditions. More specifically, we will improve the accuracy of diagnosis based on a much more extensive range of relevant factors than customarily used by clinicians and incorporated into guidelines. Undoubtedly, evidence-based diagnosis underpinned with reliable data and analytics should provide a more accurate diagnosis. It is said that clinicians can easily consider only five factors in reaching their conclusions: Machine learning systems have no such restrictions.

Solutions such as the Undiagnosed Diseases Network (UDN) may come to the rescue for individual patients and families living with the burden of undiagnosed diseases. UDN is a research study funded by the National Institutes of Health Common Fund. Its purpose is to bring together clinical and research experts across the United States to solve the most challenging medical mysteries using advanced technologies.

AI can be harnessed to minimize the patient record and presentation complexity. AI will fundamentally change medicine and healthcare: Diagnostic patient data (e.g., from ECG, EEG, or X-ray images) can be analyzed with the help of machine learning so that diseases can be detected at a very early stage based on subtle changes. AI can provide clinicians with all the information they need to make a good decision. AI algorithms can further aid in decision-making to improve the accuracy of diagnoses. By gathering data through patient interviews and tests, processing and analyzing results, and using multiple data sources, AI can come to a more accurate diagnosis. Additionally, it can determine an appropriate treatment method (often presenting options), prepare, and administer the chosen treatment method, monitor the patient during treatment, and provide aftercare follow-up appointments. This would result in more accurate diagnoses for patients and increased efficiency for healthcare professionals.

Imagine such a scenario: Before a clinician sees a patient, while the patient is still just scheduled, AI has looked at the medical history. It has reviewed the patient's chief complaint, risk factors, CT scans, ECGs, and blood tests. It may also crawl into billions of de-identified medical records, recognize correlations with your patient, and instantly establish a diagnosis suggestion.

AI does all that heavy lifting in the background, but the decision-making still rests with you. AI pulls up the most recent heart ultrasound, an echocardiogram, for you to look at. So, a 60-year-old patient presents to you for the first time but has a history of diabetes, hypertension, and hyperlipidemia with ECG abnormalities. AI, having consulted with potentially billions of anonymized patient data, will predict that the patient will need a CT for semi-urgent coronary angiography. Dr. William Schwartz published an article in the *New England Journal of Medicine*, "Medicine and the Computer," in which he speculated that computers and physicians would engage in a frequent dialogue in the future.[58] The computer continuously takes note of history, physical findings, and laboratory data, alerting the clinician to the most probable diagnosis and suggesting the appropriate, safest course of action.

AI Applications That Augment Clinical Decision Making

In recent years, several smartphone apps have been developed for doctors, allowing them to crowdsource data with their peers to facilitate diagnostic accuracy. This is accomplished by taking advantage of multiple specialists' automatic input and experience.

One app that is especially popular for sharing medical images is Figure 1. It has been downloaded over a million times and has over 100,000 active users. Figure 1 lets you share photos of skin lesions, X-rays, lab results, etc., to get a quick diagnosis from other clinicians. The app also includes a forum to ask questions about specific cases or diseases. This type of crowdsourcing can be precious for diagnosing complex cases because it allows you to draw on the expertise of multiple specialists simultaneously.

Another app that is increasingly popular among doctors is HealthTap. HealthTap allows you to ask questions about specific diseases or health problems and receive feedback from other doctors. It has 7.6 million registered members, which includes 140,000 doctors. The app also consists of a database of articles written by doctors on various health topics. This type of crowdsourcing can be valuable because it gives you access to expert opinions and first-hand experiences from people who have dealt with similar problems.

Medscape Consult, the most widely used doctor crowdsourcing app, enables doctors worldwide to help one another with difficult cases. Recently, data from Medscape Consult was published in Nature's *npj Digital Medicine*.[59] The study found that doctors who use Medscape Consult are more likely to feel confident in their ability to diagnose and treat patients. Nearly 60 percent of users said they would not have been able to make a correct diagnosis without using the app. And 80 percent of users said they were satisfied with the quality of the information provided by Medscape Consult.

These results are unsurprising when considering how comprehensive and up-to-date Medscape's content is. The app includes information on drug interactions, dosage guidelines, lab values, and more, all reviewed by experts in each field. Plus, it's constantly updated with new research so doctors can ensure they're getting the most accurate advice possible. Within two years of launch, the app had been used by a steadily growing population of 37,000 physicians from over two hundred countries and many specialties, which could rapidly turn around requests for help.

Finally, the Human Diagnosis Project, also known as Human Dx, is a web – and mobile-app-based platform that has been used by more than 6,000 doctors and trainees from forty countries. It allows users to submit photos of medical cases and their symptoms to help diagnose the illness. The app is free to download on Android and iOS devices and has received high praise from users for its easy-to-use interface and helpful diagnosis recommendations.

Final Thoughts

The benefits of doctor crowdsourcing are clear. By pooling the expertise of thousands of clinicians, it becomes much easier to find the best solution for a difficult case. There is also the potential for faster turnaround times on requests for help and greater global reach, thanks to the international nature of many doctor crowdsourcing platforms.

Some risks are associated with doctor crowdsourcing; however, these can be mitigated by taking certain precautions. For example, ensuring that the information shared through these platforms remains confidential and that patients' privacy is always protected is vital.

When we work in concert with AI, everyone becomes brilliant. A fresh clinician is catapulted into an experienced one. We can augment and improve our diagnostic skills by working in partnership with AI.

What takes an experienced, wise, and learned clinician and their patient days or weeks, even months, to put together, AI can do it faster, routinely, and all day long. The power of combining the two would be astounding. AI will make rapid and accurate diagnoses, reduce diagnostic errors, avoid unnecessary testing, and minimize medication errors and malpractice claims. And it will cut across all disciplines of medicine.

AI will augment diagnosis and judgment. This would be revolutionary and transformative. In *Deep Medicine* by Dr. Eric Topol: "With the challenge of massive and ever-increasing data and information for each individual, no less the corpus of medical publications, it is essential that we upgrade diagnosis from an art to a digital data-driven science."[60]

We owe it to our patients to properly diagnose and treat; their lives depend on it.

## CHAPTER 6

PATHOLOGY

Automated medical image diagnosis is arguably the most successful domain of medical AI applications. Medical specialties, including pathology, radiology, dermatology, and ophthalmology, rely on image-based diagnoses; they are pattern-concentrated fields. AI tools seem to perform just as well, if not better, than human clinicians at identifying features in images quickly and precisely. But more importantly, can AI replace pathologists? Let us get back to this question later. First, let's talk pathology.

The Problems

Pathology is the gold standard for the diagnosis of cancer and other diseases. The task is repetitive, time-consuming, and not easily scalable. Because of population screening programs, inordinately large numbers of breast, colon, and cervix specimens are collected, and countless lymph nodes are resected during surgery daily. This large volume of work is understandably burdensome to pathologists. And while their workload is increasing, the pathologist shortage is worsening. It is estimated that there will be a net deficit of more than 5,700 full-time equivalent pathologists by 2030.[61] Clearly, automating the assessment of tissue samples obtained by biopsy and excised lymph nodes can have a tremendous impact on the optimization of the clinical workload of pathologists and mitigate this deficit in the shortage of pathologists.

The histopathology acquisition procedure involves processing a biopsy or surgical specimen into tissue slides and staining the slides with pigments. Pathologists then interpret the slides based on visual evaluation under a microscope or a computer screen. Discrepancies among pathologists are common; the agreement level in diagnosis can be less than 40 percent.[62] Also, the interpretation error rate can be as high as 20 percent; overdiagnosis (high false positive) is typical for experienced, board-certified pathologists.

The Solutions

Pathologists diagnose and grade diseases, such as cancer and inflammatory diseases, based on various tissue features (e.g., disturbed tissue architecture, the presence or absence of specific cell characteristics, or the presence of an abundance of inflammatory cells, etc.). Moreover, some can predict the survival outcomes of cancer patients,[63] indicating the existence of rich, yet previously underutilized, information contained in the pathology slides.

This is an area where AI could provide a fast and objective evaluation of the histopathology slides and find the most optimal treatment for these patients. Using AI to analyze tissue sections is often called computational pathology (CPATH). CPATH has progressed vastly because of significant improvements in microscopic scanning devices (which enable the acquisition of whole-slide images (WSIs), computational power, and mature algorithms.

In addition to automating current diagnostic tasks, CPATH methods can support pathologists with additional information; for example, by showing the hotspots of mitotic cells in breast cancer WSIs that are required for tumor grading and treatment of patients with breast cancer. Or, as in the case of quantitative histopathology image features that are barely noticeable by the human eye, AI algorithms could flag suspicious regions or slides for inspection. Let us look at some specific examples where the utility of AI was tested in clinical trials.

AI Applications in Pathology

Prostate cancer is the most common cancer and the second leading cause of cancer death among men in the United States. In 2020, researchers from Radboud University Medical Center in the Netherlands demonstrated the potential of AI by developing a deep learning system that outperformed pathologists in determining prostate cancer aggressiveness. This study was published in *Lancet Oncology*.[64] To train the AI algorithm, the scientists collected almost 6,000 biopsies from more than 1,200 men. This was paired with the original diagnoses from the pathology reports. The algorithm was trained to interpret the biopsies like that of a pathologist and then graded them according to the Gleason grading standard. AI and fifteen pathologists were then challenged with 100 biopsies. AI performed better than ten of the fifteen pathologists. There was also a high agreement between the AI algorithm and an expert reference standard. On a group level, the AI algorithm performed equally with the pathologists with more than fifteen years of experience.

Recently, the FDA approved the Memorial Sloan Kettering Cancer Center to develop the first-ever AI pathology system.[65] This AI algorithm is called Paige Prostate, and it was designed to detect prostate cancers as an adjunct, not a replacement, to pathologist review. With Paige Prostate, pathologists digitally scan and upload biopsy slides to their computer and import them into the program, which then compares the tissue patterns against an extensive database of tissue patterns collected at the Memorial Sloan Kettering Cancer Center.

The FDA approval was granted based on a clinical study where pathologists examined 527 digitized slide images of prostate biopsies: 171 cancers and 356 benign.[66] For each slide image, each pathologist, completed two assessments, one without Paige Prostate's assistance (unassisted read) and one with Paige Prostate's assistance (assisted read). The study found that Paige Prostate improved cancer detection on individual slide images by 7.3 percent on average compared to pathologists' unassisted reads.

The algorithm looks for patterns that have been previously diagnosed as cancer. When it finds such patterns, it highlights them for the pathologists to examine, thus ensuring that they are not missed. Hence, AI functions as a diagnostic aid and, potentially, as an independent second opinion.

Another example of innovation in algorithmic pathology is cervical cancer screening. Cervical cancer is the most common cancer among women in low-and middle-income countries. The annual worldwide burden of the preventable disease cervical cancer is more than 530,000 new cases and 275,000 deaths. The majority occurs in low – and middle-income countries, where cervical cancer screening and early treatment are uncommon. Nearly 90 percent of cervical cancer cases and deaths occur in low – and middle-income countries that lack comprehensive national HPV immunization and cervical cancer screening programs.[67] Widely used in high-income countries, Pap smear screening is the gold standard. But it is expensive and challenging to implement in less-developed regions of the world, where access to prevention, screening, and treatment services is scarce. Moreover, even in developed countries, a woman diagnosed with cervical cancer is almost twice as likely to die than a woman diagnosed with breast cancer. This is an example of a global problem that's crying out for an AI solution that could revolutionize cervical cancer screening, especially in low-resource settings in low – and middle-income countries.

In a collaboration between research teams from the National Cancer Institute (NCI) and Global Good, an AI algorithm that can analyze digital images of a woman's cervix and accurately identify pre-cancerous changes was developed.[68] The scientists used more than 60,000 normal and abnormal cervical images from an NCI archive of photos collected during a cervical cancer screening study in Costa Rica in the 1990s. More than 9,400 women participated in that prospective population study, with follow-up up to 18 years. Overall, AI outperformed human experts in identifying cervical precancers; it identified precancers with greater accuracy than a human expert review or conventional cytology. "The computer analysis of the images was better at identifying precancer than a human expert reviewer of Pap tests under the microscope (cytology)," said Mark Schiffman, MD, MPH, Head of NCI's Division of Cancer Epidemiology and Genetics and senior author of the study.[68]

This AI approach, called automated visual evaluation, has the potential to be of value in low-resource settings. Healthcare workers in many low-resource, low – and middle-income countries currently use screening by visual inspection with acetic acid (VIA), where a clinician applies diluted acetic acid to the cervix and inspects the cervix with the naked eye, looking for acetowhitening, which indicates possible dysplasia or a pre-cancerous stage of growth. Because it is inexpensive and easy to perform, VIA is widely used in locations where more advanced screening methods are unavailable; however, it's generally inaccurate and leads to many false negatives.

Automated visual evaluation is easy to perform, as all one needs is a cell phone or similar camera device for cervical screening during a single visit. In addition, this approach can be achieved with minimal training, making it ideal for countries with limited health care resources, where cervical cancer is a leading cause of illness and death among women.

"When this algorithm is combined with advances in HPV vaccination, emerging HPV detection technologies, and improvements in treatment, it is conceivable that cervical cancer could be brought under control, even in low-resource settings," said Maurizio Vecchione, executive vice president of Global Good.[68] The scientists plan to further improve the algorithm by incorporating cervical images from women of different geographic regions to ensure that subtleties in the appearance of the cervix among women don't bias or affect the algorithm's accuracy.

A third example of AI's innovation in pathology is in cancers of unknown primary (CUP). In 1–2 percent of cancer cases, we cannot determine the primary site of a tumor. With a median survival of 2–16 months, the prognosis of CUP is poor, mainly because our current approach to cancer therapy relies almost entirely on identifying a primary tumor that can be targeted by therapeutics, including chemotherapy, neoadjuvant therapy, surgery, and radiation. In the lucky few patients, we can find a primary. The chase to confirm a diagnosis is expensive and diagnostically extensive; often, patients endure further workups that can include added laboratory tests, biopsies, and endoscopic procedures performed in search of the elusive alien. This also often delays the start of treatment, which is doubly awful.

To improve diagnosis for patients with complex metastatic cancers, especially those in low-resource settings, a group led by Dr. Faisal Mahmood of the Division of Computational Pathology at the Brigham and Women's Hospital and the Pathology department at Harvard Medical School developed an AI algorithm called Tumor Origin Assessment via Deep Learning (TOAD) to simultaneously identify the tumor as primary or metastatic and predict its site of origin. The researchers trained their model with WSIs of tumors from over 22,000 cancer cases, tested TOAD in about 6,500 patients with known primaries, and then challenged the algorithm with complicated metastatic cancers to establish its efficacy on CUPs. For tumors with known primary origins, the model correctly identified cancer 83 percent of the time and listed the diagnosis among its top three predictions 96 percent of the time. The researchers then tested the model on 317 CUP cases for which a differential diagnosis was assigned, finding that TOAD's diagnosis agreed with pathologists' reports 61 percent of the time and top-three agreement in 82 percent of cases. They published this study in *Nature*, one of the most prestigious scientific journals.[69]

Interestingly, TOAD's performance was comparable to genomic sequencing, both germline and somatic, to predict tumor origins, a precise but expensive last resort method to identify an unknown or rare disease or cancer. Genomic testing is not always performed for patients, especially in low-resource settings. "The top predictions from the model can accelerate diagnosis and subsequent treatment by reducing the number of ancillary tests that need to be ordered, reducing additional tissue sampling, and the overall time required to diagnose patients, which can be long and stressful," Mahmood said. "Top-three predictions can be used to guide pathologists' next steps. In low-resource settings where pathology expertise may not be available, the top prediction could potentially be used to assign a differential diagnosis. This is only the first step in using whole-slide images for AI-assisted cancer origin prediction, and it's a fascinating area with the potential to standardize and improve the diagnostic process."[69]

There are many more examples, but these are the most immediate and impactful applications of AI in pathology for clinicians not specialized in the field.

Final Thoughts

As you can see, pathology AI algorithms can be used in various ways. When ready for primetime, AI can complement pathologists. It's premature to suggest that they are ready for primetime or the more audacious claim that they can replace a pathologist altogether.

For a pathologist, a mundane task like slide-reading is still a labor-intensive process. That, and other bureaucratic tasks, seem to stretch their days out forever. Slide digitization or WSI appears to have mitigated that burden significantly. AI can be trained to process WSIs brutally efficiently, even pointing out problem areas or abnormalities much faster than a pathologist could. For instance, highlighting regions in a prostate biopsy using different colors to represent different Gleason grades.

Another example is highlighting lung cancer growth patterns by adenocarcinoma subtype using CPATH methods. AI methods such as segmentation, detection, and classification can enable the objective quantification of established biomarkers that a pathologist, and the rest of us, require in clinical practice. This will undoubtedly make pathologists more efficient, perhaps even more proficient. It should make them work *smarter* by improving their accuracy and efficiency.

There are even more ways in which AI can reduce the professional burden of pathologists, which might be a fortuitous outcome, given the current and worsening projected shortage in this profession. The overall goal is to reduce the time it takes for pathologists to do what they do so well. Three possibilities I can envision:

First, AI can screen biopsies and filter out the easy (benign) cases. The system can flag a case if the opinion differs from the pathologist's. It also can give feedback during the first read, showing the pathologist where to look. In this case, the pathologist needs only confirm the opinion of the AI system.

Second, after the pathologist's initial read, we can use AI to provide a second opinion. Merging the pathologist's expertise with the second opinion of an AI system may be the best of both worlds.

Third, mundane and tedious work in microscopy, such as quantitative grading of immunohistochemistry stains and counting mitotic figures, are plausibly better suited for AI.

The development of CPATH algorithms of increasing accuracy across many fields in pathology has been promising and has the potential to help pathologists in their clinical practice. The inimitable Dr. Topol says, "AI potentially enables pathologists to focus more cognitive resources on higher-level diagnostic and consultative takes. For example, integrating molecular morphologic and clinical information to assist in treatments and clinical management decisions for individual patients."[70] Amen, sir.

Pathologists are not likely to be replaced with AI algorithms anytime soon. I think it's a simplistic view that fails to realize the full breadth of tasks a pathologist performs. It is important to stress that a pathologist's job extends beyond simply analyzing a biopsy specimen under a microscope. Concurrent with being microscopists, they integrate their understanding of the disease. Often, they communicate and explain the unusual or abnormal findings to the other clinician or team overseeing the patient's care and correlate that with the other relevant clinical data in the patient's medical chart— the patient's unique phenotype—to arrive at a diagnosis. AI algorithms that work with pathologists rather than as stand-alone solutions could be achieved relatively soon. This is to avoid the need for tedious, repetitive work. In low – or middle-income countries, where access to pathological expertise is challenging and sometimes even impossible, algorithms could yield urgently needed data to inform diagnoses, which would be an essential step forward. The infrastructure around digital pathology in some settings, such as rural hospitals, would present challenges. We must seek creative solutions as a workaround. For example, a telepathology system could be set up so that pathologists in urban areas can consult with their colleagues in rural hospitals. The use of cloud-based storage and transmission systems could also help to overcome any bandwidth limitations. With careful planning and execution, it is possible to provide high-quality pathology services even in the world's most remote areas.

## CHAPTER 7

RADIOLOGY

There is no doubt that AI has the potential to revolutionize the field of radiology. AI-enabled tools are already used to help radiologists make diagnoses. Recent advances in AI have led to the development of deep learning neural networks that can identify pathologies in radiological images with greater accuracy than an average radiologist. For instance, AI algorithms can find pathologies in radiological images like bone fractures and potentially cancerous lesions such as breast and lung cancers. It is important to note that these systems are constantly evolving and becoming more accurate. This would be a significant advancement for the medical field and would significantly improve patient care. There's even wild speculation by some experts that AI may eventually replace radiologists altogether. While this may be some time in the future, it is clear that AI will play a significant role in radiology.

The discipline of radiology relies primarily on imaging that contains a substantial portion of the information needed to make a correct diagnosis. A year ago, I saw a man wearing a hoodie with "Radiologist Because

Badass Miracle Worker Isn't An Official Job Title" emblazoned on its front. Funny but REAL!

Radiologists are, in fact, miracle workers. They are highly trained professionals who have developed pattern recognition skills, the visual system's ability that allows them to rapidly identify abnormalities that other untrained physicians may miss easily. Hundreds of images are typically taken for one patient's disease or injury. The number of radiological images has exponentially increased over the last decade, likely more than the number of trained radiologists. Diagnostic radiologists use multiple medical-imaging modalities—the most widely used are X-ray radiography, CT, MRI, and PET scans—to detect and diagnose diseases. In each of these approaches, radiologists use a collection of images for disease screening and diagnosis, to find the cause of illness, and to monitor the patient's trajectory throughout a disease. CT, MRI, and PET scans generate hundreds of images per exam, while X-rays are usually in the single digits per exam.

The Problems

More than 800 million medical scans are performed in the US annually, amounting to about 60 billion images, or one image generated every two seconds.[71] A typical radiologist reads about 20,000 studies a year, which amounts to roughly 50–100 studies a day.[72] CTs and MRIs get the lion's share. A typical emergency room radiologist may look at as many as 200 imaging study cases daily, containing thousands of images. For instance, a lower body CT angiography study can produce 3,000 images.

Moreover, due to the volume of imagery to examine, these specialists have little time to assimilate all pertinent clinical information from patient records before interpreting the images. Inevitably, cognitive fatigue occurs—a common problem that afflicts radiologists—leading to diagnostic inaccuracies, mainly due to the sheer volume of studies a radiologist must process at any given time—massive diagnostic inaccuracy results from fatigue and overreliance on image interpretation without clinical correlations.

Imaging tests should only be ordered when there is a clear indication that they are necessary. However, most imaging tests performed are unnecessary and provide little to no benefit to the patient. The number of unnecessary radiologic tests in America is staggering. According to the Food and Drug Administration and the National Institute of Medicine, more than 30 percent of all diagnostic imaging procedures in the US are not medically necessary.[73][74] This amounts to an estimated 70 million unnecessary tests each year. The cost of these tests is also staggering, totaling more than $30 billion annually, for which taxpayers foot the bill. The most common type of unnecessary medical imaging procedure is CT scans, which account for 40 percent of all such procedures. This high rate of waste is particularly troubling given that Medicare recipients are disproportionately affected by it; they account for more than half of all unnecessary medical imaging procedures performed annually.

There are several reasons for this epidemic of over-testing. One reason is that doctors often order these tests without considering whether they are genuinely needed. Another reason is that many doctors will order tests because they fear being sued if something is missed. Others order them because they want to ensure they have ruled out all possible causes of a patient's illness. And finally, there is a great deal of financial incentive for doctors and hospitals to perform these tests since they generate significant revenue.

This overuse of radiologic testing has profound consequences for patients and the healthcare system. Exposure to unnecessary radiation can increase cancer risk and lead to other adverse health effects, such as heart disease and congenital disabilities. Additionally, many tests require injections or other invasive measures, leading to complications like infections and blood clots. And since many of these tests are duplicative, they waste valuable resources that could be used instead on preventive care or treatments for actual illnesses.

The high number of false-positive radiologic interpretations in the US is a compounding unnecessary testing problem. For example, a study in *JAMA* found that more than 50 percent of all lung cancer screenings by low-dose CT were false positives.[75] Another study by the National Cancer Institute found that out of 1,000 mammograms, about 170 will result in a false positive reading.[76] Patients are told they have cancer when they don't and are often subjected to unnecessary and invasive tests like biopsies and even incorrect treatment.

The problem is only getting worse as more people are screened for cancer. We need to find ways to reduce the number of false positives so that patients can be confident in their diagnosis and get the treatment they need without unnecessary stress or worry. The radiation exposure from these tests can also be harmful, especially if repeated often. Therefore, false-positive radiologic interpretations need to be reduced so patients can receive accurate diagnoses and appropriate treatment without unnecessary risks. False-negative radiologic interpretations in the US can also be as high as 30 percent.[77] No surprise that 31 percent of radiologists have been subjected to malpractice claims due to wrong diagnosis.[78]

Imaging and radiology are expensive, and any solution that could reduce human labor, lower costs, and improve diagnostic accuracy would benefit patients, physicians, and the healthcare system. It is a reasonable assumption that the radiological specialty is poised to benefit from systems that can read and interpret multiple images quickly, reduce unnecessary testing, and lead to more accurate interpretations and diagnoses.

The Solutions

Billions of labeled datasets (in radiology, this means images from patients who have received a definitive diagnosis of cancer, a broken bone, or other pathology) exist to train AI algorithms, as most radiology departments maintain a database of historical images in a Picture Archiving and Communication System (PACS). There are numerous examples of AI radiology applications that have reached expert-level diagnostic accuracies, for instance, heart MRI, head CT scans for detection of strokes, diagnosis of bone fractures on X-ray, the detection of lung nodules using computed tomography images, the diagnosis of pulmonary tuberculosis and common lung diseases with chest radiography, and breast-mass identification using mammography scans. Let us explore some powerful examples of these AI applications in diagnostic radiology.

Breast Cancer. Perhaps there is no better example to demonstrate diagnostic inaccuracy, unnecessary testing, inappropriate treatment, anxiety, and distress in patients than breast cancer screening using mammography. Breast cancer is the second leading cause of cancer death in women. According to the American Cancer Society, 287,000 new cases of invasive breast cancer were diagnosed, and 42,000 deaths occurred among women in the United States. Globally, there are about 2 million new cases yearly and more than half a million deaths. About 33 million screening mammograms are performed each year in the United States. The test has a false negative rate of approximately 20 percent and a false positives rate over ten years of nearly 50 percent.[79]

Google Health teamed up with Northwestern University and two British medical centers, Cancer Research Imperial Centre and Royal Surrey County Hospital, to apply AI to mammography to improve diagnostic accuracy. The study was published in the leading journal *Nature*.[80] Briefly, the scientists used labeled (diagnosis known) mammograms from about 76,000 women in Britain and 15,000 in the United States to train computers to recognize cancer. Then, they tested the algorithm on images from about 25,000 other women in Britain and 3,000 in the United States and compared the system's performance with that of six US-board-certified radiologists. AI outperformed the radiologists. Remarkably, AI beat the radiologists by reading only the most recent mammogram, while the radiologists had access to contextual information, including patient history and earlier mammograms, while reading their mammograms.

Dr. Constance Lehman from Harvard Medical School and Massachusetts General Hospital and Adam Yala of MIT developed an AI algorithm, Mirai, to predict the risk of developing breast cancer on mammography. They published the study in the journal *Science Translational Medicine*.[81]

Mirai was more accurate in predicting breast cancer risk than the existing models. When using historical patient data, 42 percent of people who went on to develop cancer in five years were flagged as high risk by the algorithm, compared with 23 percent for the best existing model. The women flagged by the algorithm were three times as likely to develop cancer; previous statistical techniques were no better than random. The algorithm was also validated on patient data from Taiwan and Sweden, suggesting that its methods are diverse and generalizable, limitations that must be overcome to ensure that algorithms are not biased.

The algorithm analyzed prior mammograms and seemed to work even when physicians did not see warning signs in those earlier scans, as breast cancer screening involves not just examining a mammogram for precursors of cancer but also collecting patient information and feeding both into a statistical model to determine the need for follow-up screening.

"What the AI tools are doing is extracting information that my eye and my brain can't," Lehman said. Lehman hopes that the AI methods she's testing can benefit people who typically receive less medical attention. "A lot of people have lived their whole lives in our healthcare system as if we were in a pandemic," she says. "They do not have access to quality care and aren't being screened."[82]

To a specialist, this is massive because, again, it can overcome our limited resources and scarcity of expertise. In Rwanda, for instance, a country of about 13 million people, there were only eleven practicing radiologists in 2015.[83] Imagine how overworked these Rwandan radiologists must be! An algorithm that could scan hundreds of images and prioritize ones to follow up on would dramatically reduce the burden on these radiologists and save lives in low-resource and developing countries.

Lung Cancer. The second application is lung cancer. With approximately 237,000 deaths in 2022 due to lung cancer, it is the most common cause of cancer death in the US.[84] The U.S. Preventive Services Task Force recommends using low-dose CT to screen for lung cancer in individuals at high risk; a reduction in mortality by 20–40 percent has been shown by low-dose CT lung cancer screening. Lung cancer survival rates increase dramatically when caught at earlier stages, but about 80 percent of lung cancers are not caught early. Although low-dose lung CTs are effective in early detection, the high false-positive rate is problematic. Over 50 percent of scans are false positives.[85]

Researchers from Northwestern University and Stanford collaborated with Google Health. They developed an AI diagnostic algorithm to help screen for lung cancer using low-dose CT scans to solve two problems: a) early detection and b) lowering the false positive rate. In a study published by *Nature Medicine* in May 2019, the AI algorithm outperformed six radiologists in diagnosing lung cancer when previous CT imaging was unavailable and performed as well as the radiologists when there was prior imaging. The algorithm was developed using 42,000 patient scans from a National Institutes of Health clinical trial. It detected 5 percent more cancers than its human counterparts and reduced false positives by 11 percent.[86]

Tuberculosis. According to the World Health Organization, tuberculosis (TB) is one of the top ten causes of death worldwide. In 2016, approximately 10.4 million people fell ill from TB, resulting in 1.8 million deaths.[87] TB can be identified on chest imaging; however, TB-prevalent areas typically lack the radiology interpretation expertise needed to screen and diagnose the disease. This initiative could help screening and evaluation efforts in TB-prevalent regions lacking access to radiologists. Researchers from Thomas Jefferson Hospital trained an AI algorithm to identify tuberculosis on chest X-rays. They used 1,007 chest X-rays of patients with and without active TB. The National Institutes of Health, the Belarus Tuberculosis Portal, and Thomas Jefferson University Hospital obtained the chest X-ray datasets. The algorithm's accuracy was tested on 150 cases with an impressive net accuracy of 96 percent.[88] The researchers concluded that this was an AI solution that could interpret radiographs for the presence of TB cost-effectively and expand the reach of early identification and treatment in developing nations.

Radiomic Signature. Radiomics is a new and promising field of medical research that could revolutionize the way doctors diagnose and treat cancer. A radiomic signature is a non-invasive radiologic-based marker that helps us diagnose cancer in a much more accurate way and can be used to diagnose any cancer. The use of AI in radiomic signatures to diagnose cancer is a relatively novel field but one that has already shown great potential. The radiomic signature is a unique feature that can be extracted from medical images, CT, or MRI scans to identify patterns in the structure of tumors. These patterns can create a "signature" for each type of tumor, even if the cancer is tiny. This signature is often hidden on an MRI or CT. Unlike a traditional biopsy which represents only a tumor sample, images reflect the entire tumor burden, providing information on each cancer lesion with a single non-invasive examination. This technology has the potential to save many lives, as it can catch cancer before it becomes too advanced. This means that we can start treatment earlier and that patients have a better chance of survival. It can also personalize each person's treatment.

Radiomics-based biomarkers have been validated in various cancers; however, whether these biomarkers can help predict clinical benefit in immunotherapy, a new wave of cancer treatments that uses the body's immune system to fight cancer cells, was an open question. As immunotherapy is expensive and potentially toxic in some patients, there is a need to identify patients who are most likely to benefit therapeutically before therapy is offered.

Trebeschi et al. used an AI-based characterization of each lesion on the pretreatment contrast-enhanced CT imaging data to develop and validate radiomic biomarkers capable of distinguishing between immunotherapy responders and non-responders. The researchers analyzed 1,055 primary and metastatic lesions from 203 patients with advanced melanoma and non-small-cell lung cancer undergoing anti-PD1 therapy. This immunotherapy-based treatment is very effective in treating many cancers, including melanoma, lung cancer, and renal cell carcinoma. Radiomic features of responders and progressive lesions were directly compared to find the differences. They concluded that the algorithm could be used as a non-invasive biomarker to predict response to cancer immunotherapy; patients with the radiomic signature were more likely to respond to immunotherapy than those without it.[89]

COVID-19. Researchers at Northwestern University developed an AI platform that detects COVID-19 by analyzing X-ray images of the lungs.[90] The team developed an AI algorithm that pitted AI against five experienced cardiothoracic fellowship-trained radiologists on 300 random chest X-rays. Each radiologist took approximately 2.5–3.5 hours to examine this set of images, whereas the AI system took about 18 minutes. Having an accuracy of 82 percent, the algorithm, called DeepCOVID-XR, outperformed the specialized thoracic radiologists, finding COVID-19 in X-rays about ten times faster and 1–6 percent more accurately. AI saved money, time, and non-specialty training. Faster, earlier detection of the highly contagious virus could potentially protect health care workers and other patients by isolating the infected patient sooner.

AI Applications in Radiology

Radiology is the trendsetter with 72 percent of all FDA-approved AI algorithms. Some applications to explore:

- Merge Healthcare
- Viz.ai
- NANOXAI
- Enlitic
- Aidoc
- DeepRadiology
- Caption Health
- RADLogics
- Imagen
- Arterys

Final Thoughts

These impressive advances in artificial intelligence have led to speculation that AI might one day replace human radiologists. Geoffrey Hinton, "the Godfather" of deep learning and one of the most celebrated scientists of our time, told a leading AI conference in Toronto in 2016, "If you work as a radiologist, you're like the coyote that's already over the edge of the cliff but hasn't yet looked down." Deep learning is so well-suited to reading images from MRIs and CT scans, he reasoned, that people should "stop training radiologists now" and that it's "just completely obvious that within five years deep learning is going to do better."

While this wild speculation has not come to pass, AI's role in the future of radiology bodes well. For now, AI holds incredible promise for rapidly and reproducibly interpreting vast amounts of medical image data. However, like other emerging technologies, radiology detection AI systems require robust clinical effectiveness evaluation before broad adoption. Clinical processes for AI-based image work are a long way from being ready for daily use. For instance, we have learned from the experience of computer-aided detection in mammography that adopting promising new technologies too quickly could be a costly mistake. Computer-aided detection was accepted and reimbursed as an adjunct to digital mammography in the early 2000s based on hype but little evidence. Later, it led to more false positives without improved cancer detection.[91] As we enter this exciting and rapidly evolving new frontier, it will be important that AI systems for radiology are validated on multiple, diverse imaging datasets representative of the populations studied. Several issues need to be considered when integrating AI into radiology workflows. First, what tasks should be delegated to AI? Task delegation is a critical issue in integrating AI into radiology workflows. Radiologists must determine which tasks can be safely delegated to machines and which require human judgment. Second, what is the best way for radiologists and AI systems to interact? Third, how will stakeholders tolerate missed cancers or false positive workups due to machine learning algorithms?

In my modest and non-radiologist opinion, radiologists do more than read and interpret images. Like others, radiology AI systems perform single tasks. The deep learning models we mentioned are trained for specific image recognition tasks (such as nodule detection on chest CT or breast cancer on a mammogram). But thousands of such detection tasks are necessary to identify all potential findings in medical images fully, and only a few of these can be done by AI today. Furthermore, the job of image interpretation encompasses only one set of tasks that radiologists perform. They also consult with other physicians on diagnosis and treatment, treat diseases (for example providing local ablative therapies), perform image-guided medical interventions (Interventional Radiology), and define the technical parameters of imaging examinations to be performed (tailored to the patient's condition), relate findings from images to other medical records and test results, discuss procedures and results with patients, and many other activities. Even in the unlikely event that AI overtook image reading and interpretation, most radiologists could redirect their focus to these other essential activities.

As autonomous vehicles are rapidly becoming a reality, medical regulation and health insurance will also have to adapt for automated image analysis to take off. Many uncertainties surround the acceptance of AI-diagnosed images by both patients and physicians. Who is responsible if an AI algorithm misses a cancer diagnosis? The physician, the hospital, the imaging technology vendor, or the data scientist who created the algorithm? Will healthcare payers reimburse for an AI diagnosis? These are just some issues that need to be addressed before automated image analysis can become commonplace. With deep learning research progressing rapidly in labs worldwide, we will likely resolve these issues in time. For instance, potentially effective use of AI would be to sort mammograms and flag those most in need of the radiologist's attention. The system may also find those that are negative so that the radiologist can read swiftly, and patients could promptly be given a clean bill of health.

It should be apparent, then, that the next time you get a mammogram or an MRI, your images are unlikely to be viewed only by an AI algorithm. Radiologists will find changes to, rather than replace, their current jobs. In many cases, these professionals will need to work with and train AI systems to be effective. The radiologist's role will change from one who looks at images to one who understands the underlying algorithms and how they can be applied to medical images. Radiologists are already using AI algorithms to help them with their diagnoses. So, they will also need to collaborate with other healthcare team members to ensure that patients receive the best possible care. Many jobs will see changes rather than replacements due to the rise of smart machines. We should embrace this rather than fear, as it represents an exciting opportunity for growth and innovation.

Despite the increasing role of AI in radiology, radiologists will continue to play a critical role in patient care. AI algorithms are exceptionally good at identifying abnormalities on screening exams. However, radiologists are still needed to order and interpret subsequent diagnostic imaging and perform image-guided tissue biopsies to confirm malignancy. It is unclear exactly how AI will support the practice of interpreting radiologists within their current workflow. Still, these nuances will be significant because a missed breast cancer on screening mammography remains the most litigious situation for medical malpractice lawsuits.

Radiologists have been using AI to help with their diagnoses for years, and the technology is only improving. Soon, AI will be able to do things humans can't, like read X-rays and CT scans more accurately than a human ever could. Dr. Isaac Kohane once remarked that AI could read 250 million radiology studies in 24 hours and do it for a mere $1000![92] By quickly scanning millions of images and prioritizing ones that need follow-up, these algorithms can help reduce the burden on doctors and other medical personnel. AI has the potential to revolutionize the way healthcare is delivered in a country like Rwanda; with shortages of doctors or other medical personnel, this could be lifesaving. With only eleven practicing radiologists, it is essential to find ways to use their time and resources efficiently. Radiology algorithms can help ensure that those in need receive prompt care.

Radiologists must adopt new skills and work processes if they want to keep their jobs. Some people might be worried about this change, but I think it's good. The productivity improvements that come with integrating AI into radiology will mean that radiologists can spend more time doing what they love: consulting with other physicians about diagnoses and treatment strategies. It also likely that providers, patients, and payers will gravitate toward the radiologists who have figured out how to work effectively alongside AI.

If you're a radiologist who's afraid of change, then you're going to be left behind in the dust. As one Medical Futurist blog post put it, the only radiologists whose jobs may be threatened are those who refuse to work with AI.[93] For further reading, I recommend AI Will Change Radiology, but It Won't Replace Radiologists.[94]

## CHAPTER 8

CARDIOLOGY

The Problems

Heart disease is the leading cause of death for men and women in the United States. Every year, cardiologists treat millions of patients with heart conditions. Coronary events are estimated to occur every 25 seconds, with death from the event occurring every minute in the United States.[95] Risk assessment is the cornerstone for primary prevention of cardiovascular disease or CVD and coronary events, particularly as the long asymptomatic latency period of coronary artery disease (CAD) provides a window of opportunity for early preventive intervention.

The Solutions

Cardiology has emerged as a significant application of AI. With many FDA-approved algorithms, cardiology is leading other medical fields in terms of the number of AI applications that have been developed and used clinically. In cardiology, machine learning can predict heart attacks, iden-tify risk factors for heart disease, and diagnose heart conditions. The use of AI in cardiology is helping to improve patient outcomes and reduce costs.

The benefits are clear: faster, more accurate patient diagnosis and treatment. In addition, using AI can help reduce costs and improve effi-ciency in the healthcare system. Many machine learning algorithms in car-diology can interpret ECGs and cardiac MRIs and quantify calcium scores on CT. The most important use of machine learning in cardiology is to predict heart disease. Machine learning has already been highly effective at predicting heart attacks, strokes, and death in patients with known cardio-vascular risk factors. Accordingly, cardiologists are beginning to develop AI models that indicate a patient's risk for heart disease and stroke years before these events happen.

For example, a 69-year-old previously fit and healthy gentleman who had never had a medical problem nor seen a doctor developed persistent 'indigestion' while skiing in Aspen, Colorado. His wife had been diagnosed with atrial fibrillation requiring a brief hospital stay, and since discharge, she had been wearing an Apple Watch. This popular wearable can obtain an ECG tracing. As his assumed indigestion wouldn't subside, he thought to use his wife's watch to get an ECG tracing to ensure his heart was OK. He did a quick check, which returned as abnormal. The watch told him to call 9-1-1 immediately. He activated 9-1-1 and was rushed into the hospital. In the ER, he was found to have ST-segment elevations and a "tombstone" pat-tern on the ECG consistent with an acute myocardial infarction; a "widow maker," to be precise. He had immediate coronary angiography and two stents deployed to traverse and revascularize his left anterior descending coronary artery (LAD) blockage. Fortunately, his life was saved, and the damage to his heart was utterly reversed. The Apple Watch saved his life.

AI-powered devices like Apple Watch and others are disrupting the classical disease paradigm, which is a fundamentally flawed approach. Usually, an otherwise typical patient is doing well and living their life but sees a clinician only when they develop signs or symptoms. They're doing well until they no longer are. Then they seek a doctor, tests are ordered, and treatments are rendered based on the results of these tests. The very first sign or symptom may be a heart attack or a stroke. It could be sudden death! And we know that latent disease can be present for decades (indicated by the gradual buildup of atherosclerosis) before someone has a myocardial infarction or a cardiac arrest. Our bodies are giving off tiny signals all the time, indicating physiologic status in the form of heart rate, heart variability, electrical signals of the heart, and changes in respiration.

If we could understand these subtle patterns and process them, we may be able to identify the disease event that is about to happen or the presence of an underlying undiagnosed illness. Hence, risk assessment is the cornerstone for primary prevention of coronary vascular disease and coronary events, particularly as the long asymptomatic latency period of CAD provides a window of opportunity for early preventive intervention. That's where such AI applications can play a role.

Suppose we could understand these subtle patterns and process them. In that case, we may be able to identify the disease event that is about to happen or the presence of an underlying undiagnosed illness. Hence, risk assessment is the cornerstone for primary prevention of coronary vascular disease and coronary events, particularly as the long asymptomatic latency period of CAD provides a window of opportunity for early preventive intervention. That's where such AI applications can play a role.

AI Applications in Cardiology

Dr. Paul Friedman, Chair of Cardiovascular Medicine at Mayo Clinic, cites an example of a patient with asymptomatic left ventricular dysfunction, which has a prevalence of approximately 3 percent. It's important to know whether one has the condition because if you knew you had it, you could take medications or, in some cases, receive a pacemaker-defibrillator.

This would prevent the onset of symptoms, lower the risk of dying, and extend both quality of life and life expectancy. Using tens of thousands of ECGs, both normal and abnormal studies diagnostic of left ventricular dysfunction, Dr. Friedman's group was able to train an AI algorithm to recognize the subtle patterns in the ECG associated with left ventricular dysfunction.[96] "And by doing so, we found that after training the convolutional neural network, someone who's coming in for a routine ECG, or someone who acquires an ECG from a wearable watch or a smartphone electrode could know it about 15 seconds," Dr. Friedman stated, "Whether or not that condition was present."[97]

AliveCor, Inc. has developed an AI-enabled portable, KardiaMobile, a smartphone-connected ECG recorder for personal use to provide information to the patient and their doctor in real-time. The user places their fingertips on a chewing gum stick-sized device for about 30 seconds, and the results are sent to the user's smartphone or other electronic devices so you can track your heart health around the clock. KardiaMobile was first introduced in 2013 and cleared by the FDA in 2014 to detect atrial fibrillation and normal sinus rhythm.[98] Patients diagnosed with a heart condition, or those at risk for one, can use this device to monitor their heart health constantly. The device sends an alert to the patient's phone if it detects any irregularities, advising them to seek medical attention as soon as possible. The app that accompanies the device can provide information about heart health and track data over time.

By 2017, the FDA had cleared the KardiaBand ECG reader as a medical device accessory to the Apple Watch.[99] KardiaBand could distinguish between atrial fibrillation and a normal heart rhythm with 93 percent sensitivity and 84 percent specificity; sensitivity increased to 99 percent with a physician review of the reading.[100] Atrial fibrillation is the most common sustained cardiac arrhythmia, affecting approximately 2 percent of the general population and up to 10 percent of people over 75. Atrial fibrillation increases the risk for stroke five-fold and is associated with significant morbidity and mortality. Most patients with atrial fibrillation are asymptomatic, making the diagnosis difficult.

KardiaBand has the potential to help save lives by detecting abnormalities early on and allowing for timely treatment interventions. It is also important because it can be used by people with no other symptoms of an irregular heartbeat. This makes it a valuable tool for screening large populations for atrial fibrillation risk factors.

In 2017, the company was conducting research with Columbia University and Mayo Clinic to determine if the KardiaBand can identify early warning signs of Long QT syndrome, a cause of sudden death, especially in young people.[101] They analyzed a dataset of 2 million ECGs linked to 4 million serum potassium values, collected over 23 years, to develop an algorithm that allows KardiaBand to diagnose hypokalemia, which is associated with Long QT syndrome, with high accuracy.

The AliveCor cardiac device also benefits doctors because it provides them with valuable data on their patients' hearts. Typically, a doctor sees their patient's one or two ECGs a year. This patient now has nearly 20 ECGs obtained by KardiaMobile per month. When that patient comes in, the doctor can see all the ECGs they've done since the last visit. Which ones are afib (atrial fibrillation)? Which are normal? What's happened to their BMI, activity, and blood pressure? This is an unprecedented view that the clinician now has for the patient whose engagement goes through the roof.

KardiaPro is a platform for doctors to monitor their patients using Kardia devices, allowing an exceptional opportunity for early detection of heart rhythm abnormalities. The platform alerts doctors when a patient's device detects an anomaly. KardiaPro also tracks patient risk factors, including weight, activity, and blood pressure, and analyzes them with AI to alert doctors to potential issues. AliveCor has recorded about 60 million ECGs. This information can help doctors make better decisions about treatment plans and allow them to track patients' progress over time. The data collected by the cardiac device can be used in research studies that may lead to new treatments for heart conditions. As of 2021, AliveCor products had been tested in about 160 clinical studies published in peer-reviewed journals.[102] This inexpensive and non-invasive device has implications for use in population screening of atrial fibrillation and other heart rhythm abnormalities. Fast Company ranked AliveCor number one in artificial intelligence in its 2018 list of the World's Most Innovative Companies.[103]

Another application of AI to identify patients who are at risk for atrial fibrillation comes from a team led by researchers at Massachusetts General Hospital (MGH), the Broad Institute of MIT and Harvard, who developed an AI algorithm to predict the risk of atrial fibrillation within the next five years, based on results from ECGs in 45,770 patients receiving primary care at MGH.[104] Next, they applied the algorithm to three large studies datasets, including 83,162 individuals. The algorithm could predict atrial fibrillation risk, independent of known risk factors. Moreover, its prediction of atrial fibrillation was enhanced when the algorithm was fed information about the known clinical risk factors, such as heart failure or stroke.

"We see a role for electrocardiogram-based artificial intelligence algorithms to assist with the identification of individuals at greatest risk for atrial fibrillation," says senior author Steven A. Lubitz, a cardiac electrophysiologist at MGH, and associate member at the Broad Institute, and associate professor of medicine at Harvard Medical School.[105]

"The algorithm could serve as a form of prescreening tool for patients who may currently be experiencing undetected atrial fibrillation, prompting clinicians to search for atrial fibrillation using longer-term cardiac rhythm monitors, which could, in turn, lead to stroke prevention measures," explains Lubitz.

Another application is in calculating coronary artery calcium (CAC) scoring. Expressed as Agatston scores, CAC scoring using CT is a powerful independent imaging biomarker of coronary atherosclerotic disease and one of the most important independent predictors of future cardiovascular events. A U.S. Preventive Services Task Force statement provided an evidence report highlighting that adding CAC to traditional risk models results in the most significant improvement in disease discrimination and risk stratification compared to other nontraditional factors (e.g., ankle-brachial index and high-sensitivity C-reactive protein).[106] However, despite the mounting evidence for its use, CAC testing remains underutilized in current clinical practice because of two significant limitations. First, CAC scoring using gated coronary CT scans, the gold standard, is often costly, prohibiting its utilization in small hospitals and low-resource countries. The second limitation to widespread adoption is that the presence of CAC is not routinely reported nor quantified on the countless routine, non-gated chest CTs for non-cardiac indications (e.g., lung cancer screening, infection, etc.). Doing so may allow the diagnosis and early intervention in millions of patients with CAD. AI-based automation of CAC scoring has the potential to address these shortcomings in current clinical practice.

Illustrating the growing potential of AI-assisted technology to enhance the detection of heart disease, Stanford and Mayo Clinic researchers demonstrated a deep-learning algorithm that can accurately, rapidly, and reliably provide rapid CAC scoring using both gated coronary calcium and routine non-gated chest CTs.[107] This model can improve efficiency and reduce potential barriers to obtaining CAC scoring in everyday clinical practice. Using such a robust algorithm could allow millions of patients at risk for cardiovascular disease to be identified and presented with the opportunity to start preventive medication and lifestyle changes to reduce the risk of myocardial infarction.

Another application in cardiology is an algorithm called CRAT (cardiac risk assessment tool). It was developed by a team of researchers at Stanford University School of Medicine. It used machine learning techniques to predict and prevent sudden cardiac death risk in patients post-myocardial infarction. The algorithm is more accurate than traditional methods such as Framingham Risk Score or SCORE (Systematic

Coronary Risk Evaluation), which are used to assess heart attack risk in people without symptoms.[108]

Another application is the calculation of the CHA2DS2-VASc Score, the most utilized method to predict thromboembolic risk in atrial fibrillation.[109] CHA2DS2 stands for (**Congestive** heart failure, **Hypertension, Age** (> 65 = 1 point, > 75 = 2 points), **Diabetes,** previous **Stroke**/transient ischemic attack (2 points). **VASc** stands for vascular disease (peripheral arterial disease, previous myocardial infarction, aortic atheroma), and sex category (female gender) is also included in this scoring system. This score helps doctors decide whether preventive measures such as anticoagulants should be prescribed.

Both CRAT and CHA2DS2-VASc scores are examples of how AI algorithms can be used effectively in cardiology diagnostics. While other algorithms may be just as good or even better than these two examples, clinicians must stay informed about the latest advances to provide their patients with the best care.

The AI interpretation of ECGs is already prevalent, and future applications are likely to aid physicians during invasive electrophysiology procedures, e.g., to make predictions from contact intracardiac electrograms or to predict the spatiotemporal patterns of activation in the myocardium. Interventional cardiology has also embraced the opportunities of AI, with applications in the identification and evaluation of coronary disease from angiograms, analysis of intravascular ultrasound, non-invasive functional assessment of coronary stenosis, and interpretation of pressure-wire pullback data.[110] This may assist physicians in performing safer angiography and improving the diagnostic accuracy of physiological evaluation of coronary stenosis.

Another algorithm could predict major adverse cardiac events (MACE) with 86 percent accuracy.[111] MACE includes things like heart attacks, strokes, and death. These results suggest that AI can help doctors better predict patient outcomes, improving care.

IBM's Medical Sieve is another example of an algorithm in cardiology, which is touted to become the next generation "cognitive assistant" with analytical reasoning capabilities and a wide range of clinical knowledge.[112] The algorithm will be qualified to assist in clinical decision-making in radiology and cardiology. Medical Sieve can scan through millions of pages in seconds and collect unlimited data from various sources that are available to clinicians, such as imaging, ECG recordings, unstructured free text, and outputs from sensors and monitors, all of which need to be interpreted to reach a diagnosis and treatment plan. It could also look up relevant medical information and keep doctors up to date in clinical research. Facilitation of analysis and interpretation of all these different data sources may enable us to deliver precision medicine; precise information on everyone's diagnosis, prognosis, and treatments. A shift from 'one-size fits all' to a more data-driven approach will identify those patients who will benefit most from specific therapies.

Final Thoughts

As technology advances, so does the field of cardiology. One such innovative advancement is the use of AI in cardiovascular disease diagnosis and treatment. It is essential to understand how AI algorithms work. These algorithms are designed to learn from data and improve over time. They can be used for various tasks, including diagnosing heart disease and predicting patient outcomes. The advantage of using AI algorithms is that they can analyze substantial amounts of data quickly and accurately. This allows them to identify patterns that would be difficult for humans to see.

The use of AI in cardiovascular research has expanded exponentially in recent years, and a few pioneering applications are already used in mainstream clinical practice. Among other benefits, AI has been deployed to interpret echocardiograms, automatically identify heart rhythms from an ECG, uniquely identify an individual using the ECG as a biometric signal and detect the presence of heart disease (such as left ventricular dysfunction) from the surface ECG. While these algorithms are still in their early stages of development, they have already shown promise in improving patient care. AI may empower primary care clinicians and non-cardiologists by providing automated ECG diagnoses that can guide decisions on whether to treat or refer for specialist cardiology care.

However, we must temper our enthusiasm a little because of the challenges in deploying AI in frontline healthcare. While there is evidence that shows the potential benefits of using AI algorithms in cardiology, more research needs to be done to determine their full impact on patients. The validity, interoperability, and generalizability of these algorithms, which are developed in controlled research settings, when it comes to the applicability to diverse real-world populations are yet unclear.

For example, it is not yet known whether these algorithms are as accurate when used in clinical practice as when tested in studies or silico. Therefore, further research is needed to determine if these algorithms can help clinicians make better diagnoses and therapy decisions for patients with cardiovascular diseases. Despite these limitations, there is no doubt that AI can signify a paradigm shift in cardiology, which has exciting potential for helping clinicians diagnose and treat cardiovascular diseases.

CHAPTER 9

DERMATOLOGY

The Problems

Skin disease is prevalent and is a leading cause of morbidity worldwide. Skin cancer is the most common cancer in the United States, and there are critical windows for timely diagnosis of these cancers that can impact mortality and morbidity. Every year there are about 5.4 million new cases of skin cancer in the United States. While the five-year survival rate for melanoma, which accounts for most skin cancer deaths, detected in its earliest stages is 99 percent, that rate plummets to 14 percent if it's diagnosed in its late stages after it spreads to lymph nodes.[113] Early detection is vital; it will save someone's life.

With relatively few practicing dermatologists in the United States, there is a growing demand for their services. Patients sometimes must wait months for an appointment, causing delays in diagnosis and treatment of this time-sensitive cancer. Consequently, most patients who suffer from skin diseases are seen by primary care clinicians.

This dermatologist shortage is especially dire in developing low-resource settings in low – and middle-income countries. This is particularly acute in countries in sub-Saharan Africa. For instance, about 30 dermatologists in Nigeria serve an estimated population of over 120 million.[114] Ethiopia is even worse; approximately 20 dermatologists practice in a nation of over 110 million people. This dermatologist shortage trend is seen elsewhere in the developing world, too.

Skin conditions are among the most common chief complaints in primary care settings, representing 15–26 percent of all doctor visits. Non-specialist clinicians are often relied upon to diagnose and treat common skin conditions like psoriasis, eczema, and acne due to the growing demand for dermatologists' services.[115] Notably, these clinicians frequently misdiagnose skin diseases up to 48 percent of the time.[116] While it is possible for a clinician without formal training in dermatology to accurately diagnose some simple cases of common skin problems using readily available online resources like medical information portals, online image search engines, and textbook images, more complex cases are often best handled by a specialist dermatologist. This suggests that, when it comes to diagnosing concerning forms of cancerous lesions on the skin, for example, dermatologists are undoubtedly more accurate.

The Solutions

Dermatologists also often complain about the lack of time with each patient due to busy clinic schedules. The use of AI technology would enable these specialists to see more patients without having to sacrifice the quality of care. Furthermore, AI would make available more convenient hours, including evenings or weekends, so that people from all walks of life could seek medical attention when needed.

The case for AI in dermatology is essential—in fact, desperately needed—to provide access to a depleted specialty and relieve the burden of misdiagnosis on non-specialist clinicians. In the absence of a dermatologist, they must step up and manage these patients. In addition, we know that dermatologists do more than examine discoloration and moles; they often treat or remove them. Like radiology and pathology, dermatology is a pattern-recognition intensive field of medicine, where AI excels. The specialty of dermatology is ripe to be disrupted, revolutionized, and transformed by AI. Dermatology indeed may be leading a paradigm shift. Let us look at some of the promising AI applications in dermatology.

AI Applications in Dermatology

AI research in dermatology is extensive. Most AI applications focus on differentiating between benign and malignant skin lesions. Here, I will present some of the most promising applications of AI tools in dermatology.

A groundbreaking study was published in *Nature* in 2017. In collaboration with Google Health, researchers at Stanford University developed an algorithm for diagnosing skin cancer using a database of nearly 130,000 skin disease images. Perhaps most striking is that an average dermatologist looks at about 200,000 in their lifetime, but it took the AI algorithm only three months to ingest 130,000 images. The algorithm not only achieved dermatologist-level accuracy in diagnosing skin malignancy but also outperformed 21 board-certified Stanford dermatologists on a set of photographic and dermoscopic images.[117] The finalized diagnostic model can be deployed on mobile devices, potentially improving the accessibility of skin-lesion screening.

In another skin cancer study, the Stanford algorithm was tested against a much larger group of 58 international dermatologists for the specific diagnosis of melanoma, and again, it outperformed most humans.[118] AI surpassed the performance of all these dermatologists. The algorithm not only missed fewer melanomas, but it was less likely to misdiagnose benign moles as malignant, the European Society for Medical Oncology found.

These AI diagnostic models can have profound implications. The digital processing of smartphone-selfie skin lesions with the proliferation of mobile apps can potentially improve the accessibility of skin-lesion screening at the expert level globally. The goals are to make smartphone app evaluation of melanoma attain a better diagnostic accuracy and achieve high sensitivity and specificity to be comparable to dermatologists.

This groundbreaking study by Google Health for assessing skin diseases[117] was expanded to answer an important question. While several algorithms have been developed to help interpret clinical and dermoscopic images for various skin conditions, an open question remains whether AI assistance can help primary care physicians and nurse practitioners diagnose skin conditions accurately.[119] As mentioned, most skin disease is seen by primary, i.e., non-dermatologist clinicians.

A recent paper published in *JAMA Network Open* demonstrated how non-specialist doctors could use AI-based tools to improve their ability to interpret skin conditions. Jain et al. hypothesized that AI could help primary care physicians (PCP) and nurse practitioners (NP) diagnose skin conditions more accurately. In this study, PCPs and NPs retrospectively reviewed 1,048 cases representing nearly 120 different skin conditions with AI assistance. Forty board-certified clinicians, including 20 PCPs; mean experience, 11.3 years and 20 NPs; mean experience, 13.1 reviewed 1048 retrospective cases, representing 120 different skin conditions. The results were self-evident; AI augmentation significantly improved the diagnostic accuracy of both the PCPs, whose accuracy went up from 48 to 58 percent and the NPs, whose accuracy increased from 46 to 58 percent.[120]

The implications of the study are impressive. Although examination of skin conditions by dermatologists results in significantly higher diagnostic accuracy and better clinical outcomes, they only see one in three patients with skin conditions. Primary care clinicians see the majority. The lack of access to dermatologists means that non-dermatologists have and will continue to play a pivotal role in assessing skin lesions and initiating clinical management and referrals. AI may help those clinicians diagnose skin conditions more accurately in primary care practices, where most skin diseases are initially seen. Appropriate diagnosis of dermatologic conditions at the point of care in primary care settings could translate to fewer delays in diagnosis and management and increased capacity for dermatology offices. AI-based tools could have an immediate and tremendous impact: AI has the potential to enhance triage and prioritize the urgency of referrals.

Google DERM ASSIST. According to Peggy Bui, M.D., product manager at Google Health, the tech giant's health and wellness division, each year, there are nearly ten billion Google Searches related to skin, nail, and hair issues.[121] While the Google Search bar is the go-to place for most people, the description of the skin condition of concern is much better enhanced by pictures rather than words alone because a picture is worth a thousand words.

Currently, the standard of care to establish a diagnosis in dermatology includes properly taking a patient's history and performing a physical examination in a well-lit examining room. In addition, a clinician assesses for texture and specific signs of a given lesion. We can then use this information to determine if additional investigations or imaging are necessary or if a biopsy is needed. By using this approach, clinicians can ensure that patients receive the most accurate diagnosis possible.

Google DermAssist is another revolutionary AI tool developed by Google Health to disrupt the standard of care in dermatology evaluation and diagnosis. Intended to be a teledermatology AI tool, the app uses as input images of the skin condition and a structured medical history. These images are taken using consumer-grade point-and-shoot cameras and mobile devices without specialized hardware. This teledermatology tool makes AI's image interpretation possible within seconds on a smart device. Such use could enable clinicians to conduct follow-up tests (e.g., potassium hydroxide test to confirm fungal infection), ask clarifying questions about the medical history, or perform a closer physical examination to realize more significant improvements in diagnostic ability. The goal is to develop an accurate, easy-to-use teledermatology tool that can provide high-quality care for more than two billion people with skin conditions who are challenged daily by limited access to dermatology.

This teledermatology app is web-based, and Google Health plans to launch it in Europe, but it's not seeking FDA approval in the US. "The tool is not intended to provide a diagnosis nor be a substitute for medical advice as many conditions require clinician review, in-person examination, or additional testing like a biopsy. Rather we hope it gives you access to authoritative information so you can make a more informed decision about your next step," Dr. Bui remarked.[121] Recently, the AI model that powers the tool passed clinical validation, and the tool has been CE marked as a Class I medical device in the European Union.

How it works is simple: Once the app is launched, one simply uses their phone's camera to take three images of the skin, hair, or nail concern from different angles. You'll then be asked questions about your skin type, how long you've had the issue, and other symptoms that help the tool narrow down the possibilities. The AI model analyzes this information and draws from its knowledge of 288 conditions to give you a list of possible matching conditions that you can research further. For each matching condition, the tool will show dermatologist-reviewed information and answers to commonly asked questions, along with similar matching images from the web. The skin image with diagnosis report can then be sent to your primary doctor, and if the lesion is urgent enough, perhaps you get seen by a dermatologist sooner. Inevitably, this is a better use of your time, your doctor's time, and the ever-too-busy specialist's time.

3Derm Systems, Inc. 3Derm is a Boston-based company that uses AI in teledermatology. DermSpot is an app that uses AI and highly standardized skin images to autonomously detect melanoma, squamous cell carcinoma, and basal cell carcinoma. This innovative technology was granted two FDA

Breakthrough Device designations, which is a testament to its tremendous potential in dermatology.[122] Hoping to bring dermatologist-level triage to primary care, DermSpot was developed in collaboration with primary care physicians and dermatologists. The AI algorithm gives primary care providers one of two actionable triage decisions: refer the patient for potential skin cancer or watchful waiting for a benign concern. Like Google DermAssist, DermSpot could revolutionize how skin cancer is detected and treated. This could save many lives by catching these cancers early on when they are most treatable.

In 2020, Digital Diagnostics purchased 3Derm Systems. For 3Derm Systems, this acquisition provides it with access to Digital Diagnostic's vast resources and expertise in AI diagnostics. Digital Diagnostics, formerly known as IDx, scored Food and Drug Administration approval for its medical device that uses AI to detect diabetic retinopathy (De Novo) without input from a doctor.[123] It was the first such device with that approval.

Other Skin Diseases. In the preceding section, we explored some AI applications that can discriminate between and accurately diagnose benign nevi vs. melanoma. These applications are typically validated by comparing AI's efficacy in correctly diagnosing benign or malignant lesions against that of board-certified dermatologists. There are also significant applications for other common skin conditions such as pressure ulcers, inflammatory skin diseases, and dermatopathology. I recommend Gomolin et al.'s comprehensive review in *Frontiers in Medicine*.[124]

Several original studies have also begun classifying non-melanoma skin cancers (also known as keratinocyte carcinomas) vs. benign and pre-malignant lesions. The Skin Cancer Foundation has estimated that there are over 3.6 million new cases of basal cell carcinoma (the most common form of non-melanoma skin cancer) and 1.8 million squamous cell carcinomas diagnosed yearly in the US.[125] While many of these tumors are still considered benign, it is essential to understand the potential implications that a diagnosis of non-melanoma skin cancer may have on your life.

Unlike melanoma, which can often be fatal if not caught early enough, non-melanoma skin cancers are typically very slow-growing and rarely spread to other body parts. However, because they can occur in areas frequently exposed to the sun (such as the face or hands), these tumors can often be quite noticeable and cause significant cosmetic concerns for those affected by them. In addition, many people do not realize that treatments for non-melanoma skin cancers (such as surgery or radiation therapy) can often be costly and time-consuming. Spyridonos et al. developed an AI model that could differentiate between actinic keratosis and normal skin, with a specificity of 89.8 percent and a sensitivity of 91.7 percent.[126]

Diabetic pressure ulcers are a significant cause of morbidity and mortality. They can develop anywhere on the body but are most common over bony prominences such as the heels, ankles, and hips. The constant pressure on these areas from sitting or lying in one position for an extended period can damage the skin and underlying tissue. People with diabetes are at increased risk for developing these ulcers, as they often have impaired sensation in their feet and other body parts, which are susceptible to prolonged pressure. Left untreated, diabetic pressure ulcers can become infected and lead to severe complications such as infection, amputation, or even death. Several studies found that image recognition software may be used to study diabetic and pressure ulcer applications, which can be challenging to diagnose accurately. The results indicate that image recognition may play a vital role in diagnosing and treating diabetic foot ulcers more quickly and effectively. This technology can potentially improve the quality of life for millions of people who suffer from chronic wounds by reducing treatment times and facilitating better patient care.

Wound measurement technology is constantly evolving and becoming more precise. This is important as it can help to improve the accuracy of wound diagnosis and treatment. Recent studies have shown that AI applications can accurately segment wounds and differentiate between different types of tissue involved. This can be extremely helpful in cases where the wound is not clearly defined or when there is uncertainty about the type of tissue involved. For example, Manohar et al. demonstrated an AI application's ability to segment the area of ill-defined ulcers with a sensitivity of 87.3 percent and specificity of 95.7 percent.[127] Mukherjee et al. have demonstrated an AI application's ability to classify granulation, slough, and necrotic tissue with 87.61 percent accuracy. This demonstration shows excellent promise for the future application of AI in this field.[128] Alderden et al. described a tool that leverages data in the electronic health records of admitted patients to predict their tendency to develop pressure ulcers.[129] Pressure ulcers are a common and costly problem for hospitalized patients. The current standard of care for preventing pressure ulcers is using clinical judgment to assess risk factors and implement preventive interventions accordingly. This approach can be time-consuming and challenging, especially when resources are limited. An AI tool that predicts patient risk for developing pressure ulcers could help clinicians allocate resources more efficiently and improve patient outcomes.

There is no doubt that AI has the potential to revolutionize how we treat inflammatory dermatoses like psoriasis. Psoriasis is a chronic autoimmune skin disease that affects an estimated 7.5 million Americans. The application of AI in dermatology may help further personalize treatment for psoriasis patients. Several original research articles have already been published on this topic, and most focus on using image recognition to improve psoriasis classification methods. For example, a study conducted by Shrivasta et al. found that several AI applications could achieve a sensitivity of 94–99.5 percent and specificity of 97–99 percent when classifying the severity of psoriasis lesions.[130]

These studies demonstrate the potential for AI to help clinicians better diagnose skin diseases and personalize treatment plans for individual patients suffering from psoriasis or any other skin condition.

Final Thoughts

AI in dermatology has the potential to augment dermatologists, allowing for faster access to more approachable doctors. This will lessen the burden of non-specialist training and provide better care for patients. Dermatologists are experts in diagnosing and treating skin conditions, but there is a shortage of dermatologists in many parts of the world. AI has the potential to help fill this gap by providing an easily accessible source of information about skin conditions. In addition, AI could help train primary care clinicians who currently see and evaluate most skin complaints to identify, treat, or appropriately refer common skin problems like acne, eczema, or psoriasis. AI could also predict how well a particular treatment will work for a patient. This would allow clinicians to personalize treatment plans based on each patient's needs. AI can also supply information on how to manage these conditions at home. This would enable dermatologists to perform surgeries or diagnose and manage complicated skin diseases, which would be especially beneficial in rural areas where fewer specialists may be available.

I believe we are still in the early periods of AI development in dermatology. As with any new technology, we need to go through a period of rigorous evaluation and testing. Only after this process is complete can we begin to see widespread adoption. There are several reasons why I think it's essential to take things slow regarding dermatology AI. Primarily, safety is our top priority as clinicians. We must ensure that any new technology is safe for our patients before using it on them. Second, these technologies are still evolving, and much more research needs to be done before the medical community can widely adopt them. Finally, as with any change, there will be some resistance from those who are comfortable with the status quo. It's important not to rush into anything but rather let the evidence guide us as we move forward with incorporating AI into our practice.

There is no doubt that artificial intelligence has the potential to revolutionize dermatology. Still, one promising area of criticism has been around the inaccuracy of AI in patients of different ethnicities or skin tones. This highlights the fact that we still have a way to go to accurately train AI with the correct input datasets and documented outcomes, so it performs as we expect it to.

There are several reasons for this lack of accuracy. First, there is a lack of diversity in training datasets, which means that algorithms do not accurately reflect the real world regarding different skin tones. Second, there is often a lack of transparency regarding how AI algorithms are practically performing, making it difficult for researchers and clinicians alike to assess and improve their accuracy.

There is also the issue of liability. If AI is relied upon and an adverse outcome ensues, is the dermatologist responsible? Or is it the company that created the algorithm? Considering these issues, a common belief is that AI will only become a guidance tool and not an absolute. In other words, it may be used to help with diagnosis or treatment options, but a human clinician will always make the final decision. This cautious approach may slow down the adoption of AI by clinicians, but it will ensure that patients are safe.

A recent survey published in *Journal of Drugs in Dermatology* found that nearly 95 percent of dermatologists are open to incorporating AI into their practices.[131] Interestingly, 81 percent of the dermatologists surveyed had not integrated AI into their practices. According to the study, dermatology areas that AI was perceived to be most beneficial were malignant skin lesions, benign skin lesions, and pigmentation disorders. In some instances, almost a third perceived AI as superior to a human provider's experience. Still, most respondents did not think AI would decrease or increase the need for dermatologists in the future.

## CHAPTER 10

OPHTHALMOLOGY

The Problems

Diabetic retinopathy is a leading cause of blindness and is a treatable disease if detected early. Despite diabetic retinopathy being preventable and treatable, one in three people in the world with diabetes (100 million of 415 million people) have diabetic retinopathy, and only half know it. The burden of diabetes is ever-growing; therefore, we're looking at more incidence of diabetic retinopathy in the future. The problem with diabetic retinopathy is inadequate access and screening to prevent blindness. In short, diabetic retinopathy is a massive public health problem.

Large-scale screening programs are needed to detect diabetic retinopathy early and prevent blindness, especially in developing countries. Unfortunately, many people do not get diagnosed due to a lack of ophthalmologists in rural areas and long screening queues. This lack of timely care leads many patients with diabetes-related vision loss to go undiagnosed until it is too late.

The gold standard for diagnosing diabetic retinopathy is the fundoscopic exam. The inside, back surface of the eye, called the fundus, is a critical part of the eye that helps it maintain shape and health. It contains the retina, the macula, and the optic disc, responsible for processing images. Damage to this area can lead to vision loss or blindness. Fundus photography is a non-invasive procedure using retinal cameras to capture retina, optic disc, and macula images. It can detect and monitor diseases such as diabetic retinopathy, glaucoma, neoplasms of the retina, and age-related macular degeneration. Clinical guidelines from the American Diabetes Association recommend diabetic retinopathy screening for diabetic patients with minimal or no retinopathy every year and more frequent examination for patients with progressing diabetic retinopathy.[132]

There is a shortage of ophthalmologic surgeons in the US, and it will only get worse. The number of available specialists is currently 18,500, but by 2025 we will need 22,000 ophthalmologic surgeons.[133] This number is only going to continue to grow. Residency programs deliver about 450 new ophthalmologists annually, while an estimated 500 to 550 ophthalmologists retire annually. That's a net loss of 50-100 doctors each year.[134] Baby Boomers are getting older and need more eye care, but not enough new doctors are trained to meet the demand. This is a severe problem that needs to be addressed.

The lack of ophthalmologists in rural America is another critical issue that requires immediate attention. According to recent data, only 0.58 ophthalmologists per 100,000 people live in rural areas, compared to 6.29 per 100,000 people living in metropolitan areas.[135] Rural areas already have a deficit in accessing prompt care. This shortage has profound consequences for the health and well-being of rural Americans.

I know. I work in a field that recruits and manages ophthalmology practices. Recruitment of new ophthalmologists is challenging for many reasons. Young eye doctors are in high demand. And because of this, they can often ask for higher salaries. With fewer private practices available, young ophthalmologists may have fewer opportunities to build career equity. As healthcare shifts towards consolidated models, many young ophthalmologists choose to work for larger healthcare entities rather than start their small practices. This shift leaves less opportunity for young ophthalmologists to become business owners and limits their earning potential.

Though it may be difficult to recruit, finding new ophthalmologists to take over the practice from their older counterparts is important. The more senior ophthalmologists can offer mentorship and guidance to the new hires and pass down their years of experience and knowledge, which will help keep the practice running smoothly for many years.

The Solutions – AI Applications in Ophthalmology

Traditionally, fundus photographs are examined and interpreted by ophthalmologists, which is challenging to scale to the millions of diabetic patients at risk of developing sight-threatening diabetic retinopathy.

A new tool may help with this task: a computer model that can predict the risk of diabetic retinopathy in a patient based only on color fundus photographs acquired at a single visit. This model was developed by Google Health in collaboration with researchers at Stanford, the University of Chicago, Moorfields Eye Hospital in England, and Sankara Nethralaya and Aravind Eye Hospitals in India, using a convolutional neural network (CNN). CNN is a type of neural network that can learn the features of an image and then recognize that image even if it is rotated, cropped, or scaled. CNNs are perfect for applications such as facial recognition or object detection. Google Health partnered with providers in India to help train a neural network for this task and obtained about 130,000 images. They also hired 54 board-certified US ophthalmologists and rendered about 880,000 diagnoses.

How it was designed was remarkable. Ophthalmologists manually reviewed more than 10,000 anonymous retina scans, rating each for the level of diabetic retinopathy present. Each scan was reviewed multiple times and was graded manually on a scale of 1 (no diabetic retinopathy signs present) to 5 (extreme signs present.) The images were then fed into an image recognition algorithm. By providing the graded images to an algorithm called automatic retinal disease assessment (ARDA), it could start understanding signs of diabetic retinopathy, just like an ophthalmologist trainee would. Once the algorithm had been trained, the results were terrific. In 2016, the scientists published a paper in the *Journal of the American Medical Association*.[136] AI was on par with ophthalmologists and able to predict the risk of developing retinopathy in people with diabetes within two years. Using only color fundus photographs, the algorithm was independent and more informative than available risk factors. Google Health has since made some improvements to the algorithm, and AI can now reach the performance level of expert humans, i.e., not just ophthalmologists but retina specialists.

The algorithm not only predicted the risk of developing retinopathy in people with diabetes within two years, but it could also predict other factors that ophthalmologists and even trained retinal specialists couldn't necessarily pick up on. It found things that you usually could not see on an eye exam: microvascular aneurysms. This is challenging because microvascular changes are not known to be detectable in color fundus photographs before the development of diabetic retinopathy.

It also predicted features that you usually would not even think of. For instance, can you imagine that by just looking at somebody's retina, you could predict their age, their gender, or their risk for cardiovascular disease? The algorithm did just that! It also predicted race, smoking status, major adverse cardiac events, HBA1C, blood pressure regulation, hepatobiliary disease, coronary calcium score, and even Alzheimer's disease from the retinal image alone; diagnoses not previously thought to be present or quantifiable in retinal photos! Features that are too subtle to be found by the human eye. And it did this with **97 percent** accuracy vs. the 50 percent, or coin flip, of a board-certified retina specialist![137][138][139] This ophthalmology moonshot development, using the retina as a window to potentially track glucose regulation, cardiovascular risk, and even neurodegenerative diseases, can have far-reaching implications for public health.

It seems that Google is proving the adage that the eyes are windows into the soul! If Google Health hasn't wowed us enough by demonstrating that unforeseen biomarkers could be recognized by simply looking at fundus images—a spectacular feat in its own right—they've upped the ante by developing an algorithm to 'see' these biomarkers in the external eye pictures (pictures of the front of the eye) and detect HBAIC, CV risk, etc. To circumvent the problem of obtaining fundus photos, which require specialized imaging equipment and a trained technician, Google Health sought to develop new disease detection or monitoring approaches that are less invasive, more accurate, cheaper, and more readily available. A groundbreaking study published in *Nature Biomedical Engineering* showed that a deep learning model could extract useful biomarkers from external eye photos and detect signs of disease.[140] For diabetic patients the model can predict the presence of diabetic retinal disease, elevated HbA1c, hyperlipidemia, and cardiovascular disease. This could have a significant impact on public health, as it would make screening much more accessible and affordable. This exciting work demonstrates the feasibility of extracting useful health-related signals from external eye photographs and has potential implications for the large and rapidly growing population of patients with diabetes or other chronic diseases.

Two other common and serious eye diseases that deserve mention are age-related macular degeneration (AMD) and glaucoma. AMD is the leading cause of visual disability among the elderly in industrialized countries. AMD is a condition that affects the central part of the retina, called the macula. This area is responsible for central vision, which allows us to see objects clearly when we look straight ahead. AMD causes damage to this area of the retina, which can lead to loss of vision or even blindness. The early detection and treatment of macular degeneration are critical for preserving sight.

Glaucoma occurs when pressure builds up inside the eye due to fluid accumulation. This pressure damages optic nerve fibers and leads to progressive vision loss over time. Early diagnosis and treatment are essential for preventing further damage and preserving sight in people with glaucoma. By 2040, worldwide cases of glaucoma are expected to increase by 50 percent to nearly 112 million.[141]

AMD and glaucoma may now be diagnosed with the help of AI. This is a significant advance in ophthalmology, as these conditions often go undetected until they have progressed to a more advanced stage. With the help of AI, doctors can now identify these diseases much earlier, which gives patients a better chance of successful treatment.[142][143]

The world's population is growing at an alarming rate, and with that growth comes an increased demand for healthcare. Dr. R. Kim, chief medical officer at Aravind Eye Hospital in Madurai, India, has stated, "We need to screen them early on when their vision is still good."[144]

However, it is not humanly possible to screen the estimated 70 million visually impaired or blind people, so new technologies must be developed to make this possible. AI is a way to provide excellent care for all these people and ensure that they have access to the treatments they need. By screening patients early, when their vision is still good, doctors can catch any potential problems and treat them before they worsen. This will help to improve the quality of life for millions of people in India and beyond.

Dr. Rajiv Raman is an ophthalmologist who believes that ARDA can be used in the primary care physician's office significantly. By screening more patients, the ophthalmologist can identify and treat those with retinopathy, thus allowing them to focus on only those who need their expertise. "Every day, I should screen 3,000 patients, which is impossible," Dr. Raman says. "So, you need a helping hand. And ARDA is my helping hand."[144]

The *Nature Medicine* paper showed that from a retina image, we could predict several cardiovascular health risk factors and your risk of a significant cardiovascular event.[140] This could help clinicians and patients alike prepare for the worst. This incredible breakthrough could lead to better preventative care for those at risk for heart disease to help them lower their chances of having a heart attack or stroke. This information is essential in assisting people in making informed decisions about their health and could save countless lives.

Perhaps diagnosing diabetic retinopathy may become as easy as checking one's vital signs, carried out by medical technicians or any operator rather than an ophthalmologist. Anyone can take images of the retina with a robotic camera that a diagnostic AI can then analyze for disease, giving a clinical decision in minutes as to whether there is or not diabetic retinopathy. Fortunately, there is now an AI algorithm that can help doctors spot diabetic retinopathy, which is more accurate than human doctors at diagnosing diabetic retinopathy. As a result, millions of diabetics could keep their vision thanks to this AI algorithm.

In April 2018, the FDA approved the first ophthalmologic device to use AI to detect more remarkable than a mild level of diabetic retinopathy.[145] The device, called IDx-DR, is a software program that uses an artificial intelligence algorithm to analyze images of the eye taken with a retinal camera called the Topcon NW400. IDx-DR can detect the presence of diabetic retinopathy in patients with diabetes. IDx-DR provides a screening decision without the need for a clinician to interpret the image or results, making it usable by healthcare providers or nurses who may not typically be involved in eye care. This is important because early detection of eye disease is key to preventing vision loss. IDx-DR can help identify patients who need further evaluation by an ophthalmologist, which means they can get the necessary treatment sooner rather than later. IDx-DR could potentially improve the early detection of diabetic retinopathy and help reduce its associated morbidity and mortality.

The FDA evaluated data from a clinical study of retinal images obtained from 900 patients with diabetes at ten primary care sites. In the study, IDx-DR was able to correctly identify the presence of more than mild diabetic retinopathy 87.4 percent of the time and correctly identify those patients who did not have more than mild diabetic retinopathy 89.5 percent of the time. There are many contraindications to using IDx-DR, including patients with a history of laser treatment, surgery, or injections in the eye. Other conditions that should prevent someone from screening by IDx-DR include having a detached retina, macular edema, proliferative diabetic retinopathy, or severe vision loss. IDx-DR is not recommended for pregnant women or those who are breastfeeding. Although this technology has come a long way, some common eye problems such as glaucoma, AMD, and cataracts will still need to be caught by a regular eye exam and should not be screened using IDx-DR.

Patients will still need to get a complete eye examination at the ages of 40 and 60 or if they have any vision symptoms (e.g., persistent vision loss, blurred vision, or floaters).

Final Thoughts

AI is already making a significant impact in ophthalmology. Ophthalmologists are using AI to diagnose eye diseases earlier and more accurately than ever before. In addition, they are using it to plan surgeries more efficiently and accurately. Ophthalmology is seeing an increased demand for services but, at the same time, is facing a shortage of practitioners. This shortfall has led to longer wait times for patients seeking appointments and has resulted in some offices turning away patients. The goal is for AI to eventually handle most aspects of patient care in the office setting. For example, using AI to delegate more routine care tasks, such as eye exams and prescribing glasses or contact lenses, to optometrists better suited for those roles due to their training. Optometrists can also be assisted by PAs and technicians who can help conduct exams and manage patient files. This can free up the surgeon's time to devote their time exclusively to surgery and complex diagnosis. This will be especially help-ful in rural areas where there are not enough doctors to meet the needs of the population, like the country of Rwanda, which has a population of 30 million and only eleven practicing ophthalmologists. Obviously, the shift toward the increased use of AI will not happen overnight; it will take many years for it to be fully implemented in all areas of ophthalmology practice.

## CHAPTER 11

MENTAL ILLNESS

M ental illness is among the most common diseases affecting the world. It can affect anyone, regardless of age, race, or gender. Mental illness includes a wide range of disorders, such as anxiety disorders, mood disorders, eating disorders, and schizophrenia. While mental illness can be debilitating and even life-threatening, it is also treatable. With early diagnosis and treatment, many people with mental illness lead healthy and productive lives.

The Problems

The nation is confronting a critical shortfall in psychiatrists and other mental health specialists, exacerbating the crisis. Nearly 40 percent of Americans live in areas designated by the federal government as having a shortage of mental health professionals.[146] More than 60 percent of US counties are without a single psychiatrist within their borders.[147] Those fortunate enough to live in areas with sufficient access to mental health services often can't afford them because many therapists don't accept insurance.

The consequences of this shortage are dire: People with untreated serious mental illness are three times more likely to be arrested, five times more likely to be incarcerated, and six times more likely to die prematurely than those who receive treatment.

The lack of accessible, affordable mental healthcare severely affects individuals, families, and society. Mental illness costs America $193 billion per year in lost productivity alone, not counting the cost of treatment or hospitalization.[148]

Many people suffer from mental illnesses and do not get their needed help. Mental illnesses are often seen as less severe than physical ones, and our country lacks mental health specialists. Instead, they go to emergency rooms or primary care clinicians for treatment. This is a problem because emergency rooms are not the best place for people with mental health issues. They are often very crowded and don't have the resources that people with mental health problems need. Primary care clinicians also aren't always equipped to deal with mental health problems. They may not have the training or the experience necessary to provide appropriate treatment. People with depression, for instance, see their primary care physicians more than five times on average annually versus fewer than three times for those without depression.[149]

Primary care clinicians see approximately 50 percent of mental illnesses.[150] However, in the primary care setting, a diagnosis of mental illness, such as depression, is often missed because of the heterogeneity and severity of its symptoms, and the fact that a visit with a primary care provider can range from discussing general wellness and prevention to managing chronic conditions and providing referrals for specialty care. In many cases, the provider has only a brief window of time to address all these issues.

Mental health clinicians are some of the best diagnosticians around. Their focus on building relationships with their patients and using all available data forms leads them to accurate diagnoses much more often than non-specialists. The psychiatric practitioner also spends more time with the patients than other clinicians. This allows them to develop a rapport which can lead to better outcomes. Patients are often more likely to share sensitive information with someone they trust, which can help the provider make an accurate diagnosis. Psychiatric practitioners also use their observational skills to watch how patients interact with others, how they respond emotionally, and how they behave physically both inside and outside of the office setting. This helps them understand not only what is going on mentally but also what might be causing any physical symptoms that are present.

To enumerate four major challenges that contribute to inadequate mental illness care where AI may offer an actionable solution:

- The shortage of mental health practitioners means less detection and accurate diagnosis.

- These clinicians are more hands-on and patient-centered in their clinical practice than most non-psychiatric practitioners, relying more on "softer" skills, including forming relationships with patients, and directly observing patient behaviors and emotions.

- Unlike other clinicians who depend mostly on quantitative data like lab results or X-rays to make a diagnosis, the psychiatric practitioner must be able to take individual mental health clinical data, often in the form of subjective and qualitative patient statements and written notes, to develop a diagnosis for the patient.

- Mental health is expensive, and many psychiatrists do not take insurance.[151]

The Solutions

AI technology offers many benefits to address these challenges. AI solutions help psychiatrists, and other mental health professionals do their jobs better by collecting and analyzing data quickly. This allows doctors to diagnose more accurately and suggest practical ways to treat patients. For instance, AI effectively identifies potential cases of depression that may have otherwise gone undiagnosed.[152] A recent study showed that an AI system correctly identified depression in 82–93 percent of cases.[153] This is significantly better than current methods used by human doctors, which only have about a 50 percent accuracy when diagnosing depression. By using machines as part of the healthcare system, we can increase diagnosis and treatment accuracy rates.

In addition, AI is more affordable than traditional therapies, sometimes by orders of magnitude. AI treatments also offer more anonymity and privacy than talking to a natural person. The inherent anonymity of AI turns out to be a positive in some instances. Patients who are often embarrassed to reveal problems to a therapist they've never met before will let down their guard with AI-powered tools. This is especially important for stigmatized conditions like social anxiety or eating disorders. Online mental health services can be lifesaving for people who would otherwise avoid getting help altogether because they don't want anyone else to know about their condition.

One study found that almost 60 percent of patients who received care from an online therapist did not disclose their issues to anyone else before seeking help from the chatbot. This suggests that people feel more comfortable discussing sensitive information with a machine than with another person face-to-face. In addition, online therapy is typically less expensive than traditional therapy sessions with a human therapist.[154] This makes it more accessible for those who need it and could lead to earlier diagnosis and treatment for mental health conditions.

The advantages of AI integration into the problem of mental illness may help optimize access and convenience, improve diagnosis, speed up treatment, and improve treatment outcomes.[149]

AI Applications in Mental Health

AI is already used in psychology in several ways, so the medical community must embrace these changes. Here are some examples of how AI is currently utilized.

Diagnosis. AI is used to diagnose mental health conditions. For example, a study published in *Nature* showed that an AI algorithm was able to diagnose depression by analyzing patients' facial expressions.[151] In one study, a computer correctly identified people with bipolar disorder 87 percent of the time, compared to 74 percent accuracy by human experts.[155] This is a massive improvement as it can help more people receive an accurate diagnosis and treatment plan. Another study found that a chatbot program was just as effective as face-to-face therapy for treating depression symptoms.[156] AI chatbots are therapy tools for people with anxiety and depression. For example, a company called Woebot has developed a chatbot that helps people with anxiety and depression by providing them with cognitive behavior therapy (CBT).

Robots have increasingly been utilized as therapists for children with autism spectrum disorder (ASD). For instance, a robot named "Nao" is effective in helping children learn social skills. Virtual Reality (VR) simulations are used as treatment tools for phobias and other anxiety disorders. VR therapy uses immersive virtual environments that allow people to experience simulations of different situations or scenarios that they might find challenging or anxiety-provoking in real life. This type of therapy effectively treats things like phobias, post-traumatic stress disorder

(PTSD), social anxiety disorder, and more. It allows people to face their fears in a safe environment without real-world consequences.

Treatment Response. AI predicts how people will respond to different treatments for mental health conditions. For example, researchers at the Hadassah-Hebrew University Medical Center have developed an algorithm to predict whether someone will respond well to antidepressant medication based on their genetic data.[157] This lets doctors and therapists personalize treatment plans for each patient, leading to better outcomes.

Monitoring Patients. AI can also be used to monitor patients' progress over time. This helps clinicians see if any changes need to be made regarding the patient's treatment plan or if they are responding well overall. It also allows clinicians to track long-term outcomes, which is essential when evaluating treatments' effectiveness.

Research. AI is also utilized for research purposes into mental health conditions. This includes learning about new treatments, identifying risk factors, and understanding how different genes influence the development of mental illness.[158] For example, the Harvard Department of Psychology uses cutting-edge research to identify subgroups with clinically and biologically distinct profiles. By using brain-based measures such as cognition, neuro-imaging, genetics, and more, the researchers hope to get a complete picture of each patient's illness and trajectory. Ultimately, this research will help us improve our understanding of psychiatric illness and find new ways to treat it effectively.[159]

Risk Prediction and Intervention. Social media has had a profound impact on the way we communicate and share information. But what if this powerful technology could also be used to detect and predict mental health problems in users? Studies have demonstrated that using social media data has the potential to detect users with mental health problems. For example, the University of Pennsylvania has successfully linked Facebook data with EHRs for research purposes.[160] This study provided compelling evidence that Facebook content can be used to predict future occurrences of depression. The Facebook language users shared included references to typical symptoms of depression, such as sadness, loneliness, hostility, rumination, and increased self-reference. This suggests that an analysis of social media data could be used to screen consenting individuals for depression before they exhibit any symptoms. This could lead to earlier diagnosis and treatment, which would improve the chances of a successful recovery. While the use of social media data for this purpose is still in its early stages, it is possible that such screenings could become routine in the future.

Social media can also be a powerful tool for measuring the overall mood of a community and its impact on public health. Another study by the University of Pennsylvania showed that communities where people tweeted more about hostility, hatred, and fatigue, were also more likely to have higher rates of heart disease.[161] On the other hand, regions where tweets were more optimistic seemed to have lower rates of heart disease. "The single most predictive feature—the single word predictor of heart disease—is hate," Eichstaedt said. "You couldn't make this up."[162]

This research is necessary because it shows that online communication can help identify potential health concerns in a community and may lead to interventions that could improve public health. Machine learning can predict suicide risk by analyzing data from social media posts, emails, phone calls, or other forms of communication. By analyzing this data, machine learning algorithms can identify specific patterns that may indicate someone is at risk for suicide. This helps provide intervention before it is too late.

Veterans account for a disproportionately high number of suicides in the United States. The most recent estimates suggest that an average of 20 veterans die by suicide each day in the United States, representing almost 14 percent of all US suicide deaths among individuals ages 18 and older, which is substantially higher than expected given that veterans make up 7 percent of the population.[163] The Veterans Health Administration has recognized the severity of this issue. It has started using predictive modeling to identify veterans at high risk for suicide so they can be given targeted care.[164] This is an important step in helping to prevent more veteran suicides.

Using AI to analyze only electronic medical records of 6,360 veterans who had died by suicide between 2009–2011, researchers from Harvard Medical School developed a suicide risk algorithm. The AI model was then applied to over 3,000 suicide cases and more than one million controls. The AI algorithm was able to predict suicide risk in at-risk veterans accurately. Remarkably, most of them would not have been clinically flagged as at risk for suicide.[165]

Another study aimed to use AI to evaluate the utility of The Minnesota Multiphasic Personality Inventory-2 (MMPI-2), one of the most widely used objective personality tests worldwide and the most frequently used scale for evaluating psychopathology and emotional function in assessing suicidal risk.[166] The study confirmed that machine learning using MMPI-2 could assist suicide prevention by classifying and predicting high suicidal risk.

Education. Finally, AI is helping to provide education and training on mental health issues. For example, the website Mental Health America has produced AI that has been used in psychology for many years, and there are countless examples of its success.

Dr. Bot

Chatbots are computer programs that simulate human conversation through text or a voice-enabled AI interface. Chatbots assess mental health symptoms by conversing with a person about their feelings and emotions. The chatbot then records the conversation and sends it to a psychologist who can analyze the data to see if there are any concerning patterns.

Psychiatric signs, symptoms, and diagnoses can be extracted from audiovisual patterns, such as overall appearance, hygiene, body movement, facial expression, eye gaze, eye contact with others, speed of speech, voice volume, and short or lack of answers to questions. These bots can diagnose individuals who might be struggling with substance abuse, depression, or anxiety and provide access to convenient and cost-effective care.

The University of Southern California (USC) has developed a virtual therapist named Ellie, initially designed to determine whether veterans returning from deployment might need therapy. In a study of veterans who had returned from Afghanistan, Ellie exceeded the Post-Deployment Health Assessment administered by the military in predicting PTSD. This is an impactful solution to a problem affecting nearly 20 percent of veterans, many of whom die by suicide.[167] Veterans are one group that can significantly benefit from using Ellie as it is more accurate than traditional methods in predicting PTSD. However, this technology can be used by anyone who needs it, not just those who have served in the military. One reason that Ellie may be more effective than traditional assessments is that it can provide anonymity and privacy for those reluctant to seek help. Additionally, its artificial intelligence allows it to learn about each veteran and provide tailored support. It can also monitor symptoms over time and give feedback on how well treatments work.

Ellie appears on computer monitors and leads a person through initial questions. Ellie is far more than the usual chatbot; it can detect nonverbal cues and respond accordingly. For instance, it has learned when to nod approvingly or perhaps utter a well-placed "hmmm" to encourage patients to be more forthcoming.

Ellie makes eye contact, nods, and uses hand gestures like a human therapist. It pauses if the person gives a short answer, pushing them to say more. "After the first or second question, you kind of forget that it's a robot," said a West Point cadet helping test the program.[168]

Ellie does not diagnose or treat. Instead, human therapists use recordings of the sessions to help determine what the patient might need. Ellie observes 66 points on the patient's face and notes the patient's speech rate and the length of pauses before answering questions. Ellie can detect depression by analyzing people's facial expressions and mannerisms. When you smile at Ellie, it compares your smile with a database of controls made up of civilians and military veterans. Depression can have many different effects on people, including how they speak. People with depression often don't move their muscles of speech as much as those who aren't depressed, which results in them pronouncing their vowel sounds more clearly. This is because the muscles that control speech produce movement and sound, so when they're not used as often, the sounds they make are more pronounced.

The team that developed Ellie also has put together a newer AI-based program to help students manage stress and stay healthy. Ask Ari is an AI chatbot developed at USC to give students easy access to advice on coping with stress, dealing with loneliness, getting better sleep, or handling other complications that crop up in college life. Ari does not replace a therapist, but its designers say it will connect students through their phones or laptops to reliable help whenever they need it.

Commercially Available AI-Based Mental Health Applications

Clinicians should be aware of the benefits the following AI-based mental health apps can provide to their patients.

Happify is an effective tool for improving mental health. The app has a unique approach using interactive activities and games led by a digital AI coach, Anna. Lately, the app introduced 'adherence fidelity' into Anna, which helps users stay adherent to the activity goals they set for themselves. This feature uses natural language processing to detect when users are slipping away from their goals and gently guide them back on track.

Wysa. With the pandemic sweeping the world, many people struggle with anxiety and depression. Wysa is an AI-based chatbot that can provide support during these challenging times. The app has been trained using 100-million conversations, so it understands user input well. It offers research-backed techniques like CBT, dialectical behavioral therapy (DBT), and meditation support to help people with mental health needs. And best of all, Wysa is free to use until we get through this pandemic.

Elomia is an AI-driven therapy chatbot, predominantly working via Facebook Messenger, which acts as a companion to help people struggling with anxiety and sadness. Psychologists have developed the app to understand what one is saying and build a conversation to help the users feel better using CBT. The app is a medium to help people who can't see a therapist or must self-isolate, making the situation a bit more bearable.

BioBase. Used more by enterprises than individuals, the BioBase app collects data from a wearable device called BioBeam. The real-time data is analyzed using AI. This helps monitor one's mental well-being and physical health to provide live feedback and insights. The app reduced the average length of absences at a workplace by 31 percent and stress-related work absences to zero. An enterprise would benefit significantly from having its employees use this app to reduce stress levels and improve productivity.

Ginger.io. The AI app collects user's behavioral data in terms of the duration of their talking, sleeping, or exercising to get clues on the person's mental health. The app has been shown to help users with symptoms of depression, and it provides a viable alternative for those who cannot or do not want to receive traditional therapy. It can help specialists track patients' progress, identify times of crisis, and develop individualized care plans. In a year-long survey of Ginger users, 72 percent reported clinically significant improvements in symptoms of depression.

Each of these examples shows how artificial intelligence can be helpful in psychology. This technology has great potential for helping us better understand and treat mental health conditions.

Final Thoughts

Mental illness is a severe public health problem that can lead to disability, unemployment, and suicide. Mental illness is also one of the most difficult diseases to treat. However, with the advent of AI, mental health may finally get the attention it deserves. AI has already been shown to be incredibly effective in diagnosing mental illness, and there is no doubt that it will play a significant role in treatment in the future. The use of artificial intelligence has the potential to revolutionize mental health care by making it both more accessible and affordable. AI may help diagnose mental health issues earlier and more accurately than humans can, leading to better patient outcomes.

Clinicians should be wary of new digitization tools in healthcare due to the risks they pose to patient privacy. Healthcare has become a prime target for hackers as more and more records have been digitized. However, hacking claims data is one thing; getting access to each patient's most intimate details presents a new risk. Mainly when those details are linked to consumer data and social media logins, providers must design their solutions by employing mitigation techniques such as storing minimal personally identifiable data, regularly deleting session transcripts following analysis, and encrypting data on the server itself (not just communications). By taking these precautions, clinicians can protect their patients' privacy.

AI vendors must also deal with the acknowledged limitations of AI, such as a tendency for machine learning to discriminate based on race, gender, or age. However, these concerns can be addressed through careful design and implementation. For example, we can reduce the likelihood of bias creeping in by ensuring that data is thoroughly cleaned and labeled before training models. Additionally, incorporating feedback from human experts can help to prevent unwanted outcomes. This way, we can use AI technology to benefit everyone, regardless of their background or identity.

While there are some concerns about the safety of using AI in this area, if appropriate safeguards are in place, there is no reason to believe that AI cannot play an invaluable and transformative role in helping treat mental illness.

## CHAPTER 12

GASTROENTEROLOGY

Gastrointestinal (GI) doctors rely heavily on visual data from endoscopies and imaging modalities such as CT scans, ultrasound, MRI, and histopathology, which also play a vital role in diagnostics. Most of these modalities rely on the provider's expertise in interpreting these images. In essence, like pathologists, radiologists, and dermatologists, we are heavy on "pattern recognition." As we have seen previously with other medical subspecialties that are image-intensive, the human eye may miss portions of the image that contain the specific abnormality. This, however, is not a problem with AI since each pixel of an image in each frame of a video is analyzed, and a well-trained algorithm will not miss any such anomaly. Hence, AI has the potential to revolutionize the field of GI diagnostics similarly. The use of AI in gastroenterology is rapidly growing. AI is incredibly effective in diagnosing and treating a variety of GI conditions. Its ability to quickly analyze substantial amounts of data allows it to make accurate diagnoses that would otherwise be challenging for human doctors.

The Problems

Colorectal cancer (CRC) is the second leading cause of cancer death worldwide. Approximately 4.4 percent of men and 4.1 percent of women will be diagnosed with CRC in their lifetime.[169] Colonoscopy is the gold standard of screening modalities for colorectal cancer due to its ability to view the entire colon and detect and remove polyps during the same procedure. Polyps are small, mole-like growths that can develop on the colon lining and may become cancerous over time. The entire point of a screening colonoscopy is to detect these polyps early before they can turn into cancer.

Nearly 17 million colonoscopies are performed each year in the United States.[170] However, colonoscopy is imperfect. Even in expert hands, and when the most rigorous quality standards are followed, we can miss up to 30 percent of polyps during a colonoscopy. Some of these polyps are pre-cancerous or adenomatous. Next, I will show you how AI augmentation may help us reduce this polyp miss rate.

The Solutions

A short digression here might be helpful. Implementing AI into colonoscopy employs computer-aided detection (CADe) systems, which have existed for many decades. The year was 2003 when I first started doing CADe research in colonoscopy. I didn't at the time know that I was doing AI research! I was approached by a company that did research for NASA and had developed technology (CADe) that enabled a fighter jet traveling at 300 mph to spot a submarine from 30,000 feet away. To use this technology for benevolent purposes, the company sought to explore medical applications in diagnosing cervical cancer, a pervasive disease, as I discussed earlier, especially in developing countries. Upon receiving positive results on cervical cancer screening, the company approached me to help adapt the CADe technology to colon cancer screening in real-time during a colonoscopy.

Our research found we could train a CADe system to identify colorectal polyps in endoscopy images and videos. The algorithm recognized patterns and complex relations within the datasets. The system learned to predict outcomes, such as identifying polyps and other mucosal abnormalities. The results of our preliminary research were promising and reinforced the use of CADe in diagnostic support to gastroenterologists by locating polyps during a colonoscopy.[171]

Fast forward to twenty years later. The technology has evolved prodigiously, impressively. In addition to CADe systems for detecting polyps, computer-aided diagnosis (CADx) systems are now available to learn to differentiate the polyp's histology to characterize a polyp as an adenoma or pre-cancerous versus a hyperplastic or benign polyp. The move toward building and refining AI systems for this task was swift. Multiple approaches for CADe of polyps in live colonoscopies have been shown to improve the adenoma detection rate (ADR), an endoscopist's most reliable quality benchmark for colonoscopy performance.

Using CADe can help even experienced endoscopists achieve improved ADRs. In the AID-1 study, six expert endoscopists achieved an ADR of 54.8 percent using CADe, compared to 40.4 percent without it.[172] This improvement is likely due to the ability of CADe to learn from and adapt its calculations based on individual endoscopist performance. The use of AI to aid colonoscopy also improved the detection of adenomas in the hands of non-expert endoscopists by 22 percent, versus conventional colonoscopy, according to a study presented at the 2021 virtual Digestive Disease Week.[173] The AID-2 study evaluated the benefit of incorporating a CADe system compared with unaided conventional colonoscopy during 660 colonoscopies performed by ten endoscopists who had done less than 2,000 colonoscopies (less experienced endoscopists) each. There was no difference between the groups in withdrawal time or resection of non-neoplastic lesions, suggesting the addition of CADe had no adverse effect on the procedure. When pooling these data with those from the previous AID-1 study, it appears that the use of AI improved ADR, regardless of the endoscopist's experience. Additionally, the study suggested that CADe did not lead to longer surgery times and more tissue resected than necessary, two events that may be potentially harmful to patients. As such, this technology will likely play an increasingly vital role in colorectal cancer screening in the future.

AI also has the potential to help endoscopists maintain a consistent level of procedure quality throughout the day. Repeated tasks, such as those involved in endoscopy, can lead to a lack of focus and decreased performance over time. For instance, a study from Germany (reported at United European Gastroenterology Week 2021) showed that, without the assistance of AI, the ADR peaked between 9 and 11 a.m., at 3.5 adenomas per patient, dropped to an average of 1.8 by noon, and continued at that level for the entire day.[174] When AI was employed, the ADR remained more consistent throughout the day. AI's vigilance is the same at 1:00 a.m. as at 8:00 a.m. AI can help endoscopists maintain a consistent level of procedure quality throughout the day, correcting the human tendency to tire and lose focus with repetitive tasks.

In April 2021, the FDA approved the GI Genius™ (Medtronic) as the first CADe system for real-time detection of colorectal polyps to be marketed and used in clinical practice.[175] The approval of this system brings the realistic prospect of change in endoscopy practices for colonoscopy and other procedures soon.

The next step is to improve polyp characterization with CADx systems. Using AI imaging analysis in colonoscopy can enhance the detection and differentiation of neoplastic lesions. A negative predictive value of more than 90 percent was proposed by the American Society of Gastrointestinal Endoscopy Preservation and Incorporation of Valuable Endoscopic Innovations (PIVI) initiative as a threshold to leave non-neoplastic polyps in place without resection.[176] CADx systems for real-time polyp classification are new and innovative technologies that can help improve the accuracy of a colon cancer diagnosis. These systems use computer algorithms that analyze images of colon polyps to identify those likely to be cancerous or pre-cancerous.

My colleagues at VA Boston Healthcare System and Boston University, Drs. Satish Singh, Eladio Rodriguez-Diaz, and others have published several studies showing that AI has high accuracy in histologic prediction. They used a technique called elastic-scattering spectroscopy (ESS) and showed that it's a viable endoscopic platform for real-time polyp histology.[177] Some AI systems have performed significantly better than non-expert endoscopists. Several other studies have also found CADx systems to have good accuracy when predicting adenomatous versus hyperplastic histology of polyps, compared with the pathology-confirmed diagnoses.[178] Although these results are promising, these systems must prove capable of real-time evaluation during live colonoscopy. CADx systems are accurate and can provide results in seconds. I believe this is an excellent proposal and recommend adopting it as a procedure.

There are several reasons why we should adopt CADx. First, this technology could help endoscopists make more informed real-time decisions about treatment. It could lead to earlier diagnosis and treatment of pre-cancerous and cancerous lesions, potentially saving lives. Second, more than 90 percent negative predictive value would ensure that only patients with truly benign polyps would avoid polypectomy. Ostensibly, this could minimize the number of unnecessary biopsies and polypectomies performed each year and spare patients from the risks associated with biopsy or polypectomy, which can include infection, perforation, and blood loss. This is particularly true in patients on anticoagulation (blood thinner medications that help reduce stroke risk), whose risk of post-polypectomy bleeding is higher than average. On the other hand, stopping anticoagulation in such patients may also increase their clotting risk—the problem anticoagulation was intended to solve in the first place—potentially leading to otherwise avoidable cardiovascular events.

Finally, adopting CADx would improve patient outcomes and reduce healthcare costs by lessening the number of ER and hospital admissions due to unnecessary complications associated with biopsies and polypectomies of benign lesions.

Role of AI in Gastrointestinal Pathology

The advent of AI has proven to be very helpful for clinicians in making diagnoses, providing treatment, and predicting outcomes, especially regarding GI pathologies. Can we use AI as our primary means of diagnosing Barrett's neoplasia, esophageal carcinoma, Gastroesophageal reflux disease (GERD), and abnormal interpapillary capillary loops (early signs of GERD) based on patient responses to standard symptom questionnaires?

A metanalysis by Visaggi et al. found that AI had a sensitivity of 89 percent and a specificity of 86 percent for the diagnosis of Barrett's esophagus,[179] a pre-cancerous condition in which the cells that line the esophagus are replaced by abnormal cells. These abnormal cells can become cancerous over time. This condition is more common in people who are obese or have chronic heartburn. This indicates that AI is an accurate and effective diagnostic tool for these conditions and can be used to help endoscopists make a diagnosis. Furthermore, the study found that AI had 94 percent sensitivity and specificity in detecting abnormal intrapapillary capillary loops. This suggests that AI can be used to detect early signs of GERD. Lastly, the study found that AI correctly diagnosed GERD in 97 percent of patients who responded to standard symptom questionnaires, indicating that AI can help identify patterns in patient data that human clinicians may not detect. This means that gastroenterologists can rely on AI to diagnose patients experiencing symptoms related to these diseases accurately. This could help gastroenterologists diagnose esophageal disease quicker and more accurately than they would be able to do on their own.

Esophageal Cancer. Esophageal cancer is highly aggressive with an abysmal prognosis in its advanced stages. A study by the National Cancer Institute found that the 5-year survival rate for patients with esophageal cancer is only 17 percent.[180] However, if the cancer is caught in its early stages, the 5-year survival rate jumps to 56 percent. Despite the poor prognosis, early diagnosis and treatment of esophageal cancer offer patients a better chance for long-term survival. The gold standard for detecting esophageal cancer is esophagogastroduodenoscopy (EGD), but endoscopists can easily overlook these lesions, especially in white-light imaging. AI systems can play a significant role in detecting these cancers early by analyzing endoscopic images and biopsy specimens and looking for specific patterns that indicate the presence of dysplasia or cancer.

There is enormous potential for using AI systems to diagnose esophageal cancer, including squamous cell carcinoma and adenocarcinoma. AI systems have proven to be very accurate in diagnosing esophageal cancers. Visaggi et al. found that AI had a sensitivity and specificity of 89-93 percent and 90 percent, respectively, in diagnosing esophageal cancer.[179] In one systematic review, the performance of an AI system was equal to that of humans in diagnosing esophageal cancer from endoscopic images.[181] These results show we can use AI systems to diagnose esophageal cancer with high accuracy, often performing comparably or better than expert endoscopists.

Inflammatory Bowel Disease. In recent years, with the increasing incidence of inflammatory bowel disease (IBD), seeking more accurate diagnostic tools for IBD has become a hot topic. Currently, there is no gold standard for diagnosing IBD. A recent study examined how well 58 gastroenterologists could agree on the mucosal healing of patients with ulcerative colitis (UC) and the postoperative scores of patients with Crohn's disease (CD). The study found a limited agreement between the diagnostic impressions of different gastroenterologists. This means that if you go to see another gastroenterologist for a second opinion, they may disagree with the first diagnosis. This can be frustrating and confusing, and it could potentially lead to you not getting the treatment you need, or even worse, being given the wrong treatment.[182]

Utilizing a CADe system to analyze the endoscopic images revealed that, in addition to achieving higher sensitivity, specificity, and accuracy, the CADe systems have some advantages over traditional imaging, such as providing more comprehensive imaging information, implementing an automatic selection of the region of interest, and better reproducibility. Based on the data from 187 patients with UC, a study collected 525 validation sets from 100 patients and utilized the 12,900 endoscopic images of the remaining 87 patients to develop the CADe system. The biopsy samples marked all endoscopic images with their histological assessment. The CADe system autonomously identified microscopic inflammation in patients with UC with 74 percent diagnostic sensitivity, 97 percent specificity, and 91 percent accuracy.[183]

Ulcerative Colitis. UC is a debilitating inflammatory bowel disease that can cause recurrent and unpredictable episodes of inflammation in the colon. Episodes of relapse and remission characterize it. Identifying people with UC who are most likely to experience a relapse in their disease activity is vital for timely intervention and treatment. Gastroenterologists have long sought to develop a reliable method for predicting when patients are most likely to experience a relapse, but up until now, no such tool has existed. Currently, disease predictions are based on histologic evaluations, with histologically active disease defined as a Geboes score greater than 3 in at least one segment of the colon and histologic healing defined as a Geboes score of 3 or lower in all analyzed colonic segments.

A new study has found that AI is just as accurate as a histology-based prediction in identifying people at risk for ulcerative colitis risk of relapse. Moreover, the AI can do so in real-time, making it a precious tool for doctors.[184] This study provides hope that we may soon have an "on-the-spot" reliable way of preventing ulcerative colitis relapses.

Another study found that AI could diagnose Crohn's disease with 89 percent accuracy, while human doctors were only able to do so with 58 percent accuracy.[185]

Treatment. The development of new biologics and small molecules such as anti-TNF agents has caused a paradigm shift in how we treat IBD. With a better understanding of the IBD pathophysiology, new treatment options have become increasingly available, including anti-cytokine agents, anti-adhesion molecules, fecal microbiota transplantation, and mesenchymal stem cell therapy. Although some patients respond well to these treatments, others do not. Clinical decisions are more complex, not only for patients but also for clinicians. New treatment options are constantly being developed, and clinicians must decide which of these to use in their patients. The most critical factor in making this decision is the effectiveness of the treatment. If therapy can achieve the desired results, a clinician is likelier to use it. Furthermore, tolerability is also an important consideration. If a patient cannot tolerate treatment due to side effects, it will not be effective. Clinicians must weigh all these factors when deciding which novel treatment option to use in their patients.

Many difficulties remain to be solved in optimizing treatment strategies, improving long-term prognosis, and changing the life cycle of IBD. The lack of biomarkers that predict which patients will respond to a particular therapy and who is at risk for developing severe complications hampers our ability to make rational clinical decisions about optimal management strategies for individual patients with IBD. In addition, current therapies do not consistently achieve remission or induce durable responses in all patients with IBD. Furthermore, there is still much unknown about the pathogenesis of these diseases and how best to target interventions to improve outcomes. AI research is needed to determine which patients will benefit from each treatment and further enhance the efficacy and safety of these therapies. AI can be a valuable tool for predicting the effectiveness of certain medications. AI is feasible because of its ability to extract vast amounts of information from existing medical records and digital images to predict which biologic agent would be best to treat a given patient, i.e., a personalized therapeutic intervention. In addition, using machine learning for these purposes can help reduce costs and improve healthcare efficiency.[186]

Pancreatitis and Pancreatic Cancer. AI can also help treat GI conditions more effectively than humans can. For example, one study showed that AI-based applications might improve the prediction of disease severity, complications, and mortality in patients with acute pancreatitis.[187] The reduction in stay time leads not only to cost savings for hospitals but also shorter wait times for other patients who need treatment beds at those hospitals. In addition, machine learning algorithms are better than humans at predicting patient outcomes after surgery; vital information when deciding how best to treat a patient surgically.

AI may even be beneficial in the early detection of pancreatic cancer—a grim disease with a high mortality rate—with the 5-year survival rate at approximately 10 percent, despite extensive research efforts toward improving diagnosis.[188] Pancreatic cancer is currently the fourth leading cause of cancer death in the United States, but it is on track to become the number two cancer killer within the next decade. Several risk factors for pancreatic cancer exist, including smoking, obesity, and diabetes. However, most cases of pancreatic cancer occur in people who do not have any known risk factors. This deadly disease can often go undetected until it is too late because there are few early warning signs. The symptoms of pancreatic cancer – such as abdominal pain and weight loss – often do not appear until the disease is quite advanced. By that time, treatment may not be an option anymore. However, if pancreatic cancer is caught early enough, there are treatments available that can extend a patient's life by years or even decades. There are many reasons why pancreatic cancer has one of the highest mortality rates of all cancers. One reason may be that there are no effective screening tests for early detection, like those used for other common cancers like breast, colon, or prostate cancer. This is where AI may come in handy.

Several promising AI-based screening tools currently in development could help detect pancreatic cancer at an early stage when it is still treatable. For example, the Pancreatic Cancer Collective has funded two teams to use AI to screen for pancreatic cancer. The first team, led by Chris Sander at the Dana-Farber Cancer Institute and Regina Barzilay of MIT, is using AI algorithms to analyze large data sets from the EHR and images of the pancreas taken during an MRI or CT scan to create models that can accurately predict the risk of developing pancreatic cancer years in advance of our current methods of detection. The second team, led by Dr. Eugene Koay of MD Anderson Cancer Center, is working on a project that uses machine learning algorithms to analyze genomic data from tumors and blood samples collected from patients with pancreatic cancer. They aim to develop an AI model that can identify biomarkers in people predisposed genetically or immunologically to the disease. These biomarkers could potentially be used as part of a screening test one day to identify at-risk individuals.[188]

Recently, researchers from Mayo Clinic showed that radiomics-based machine-learning models could detect pancreatic cancer up to three years before it is clinically diagnosed.[189]

Cirrhosis. Can you imagine using an ECG to diagnose cirrhosis? I mean, wow! How often is the diagnosis of cirrhosis missed when a patient presents to the ER, sometimes even upon a presentation with a severe upper GI bleed?

Cirrhosis of the liver is a serious and potentially fatal disease that affects millions of people each year. A new study has created a fully automated method of non-invasively detecting cirrhosis and measuring its severity using an AI-based model. The study published in the *American Journal of Gastroenterology* found that abnormalities in ECGs can be used to detect cirrhosis. The AI neural network was trained and then validated on a conventional 12-lead ECG that analyzed heart rhythms from 4,197 patients with cirrhosis within one year of liver transplant and 16,730 age – and sex-matched controls.[190]

With sensitivity and specificity of over 83 percent, the study's results showed that the AI-based model could be used to screen for cirrhosis in at-risk populations or as part of routine health screenings. The potential benefits of this approach are enormous, as early detection could lead to earlier treatment and improved outcomes for patients with cirrhosis.

"In the subset of patients with serial ECGs obtained years before and after liver transplant, the ACE scores closely mirrored the progression and resolution of the disease, increasing over time until transplant and rapidly dropping to very low levels after transplant," said the lead researcher, Dr. Ahn.[191]

Capsule Endoscopy. AI has the potential to play a more significant role than others in specific procedures. One such procedure is wireless capsule endoscopy. This involves swallowing a capsule equipped with a camera. The camera captures images as it passes through the GI tract. These images are then downloaded and studied by a gastroenterologist.

This procedure does not rely on the gastroenterologist's skill but rather their ability to detect an anomaly in video images. It also captures a large amount of data for a single patient, which can be exhaustive for the gastroenterologist to review. By automating the interpretation of the images from a wireless capsule endoscopy, we can make the process much more efficient. An efficient hypothetical model would be AI flagging likely abnormal studies and prioritizing them over those that appear normal for the human interpreter.

Final Thoughts

AI represents a monumental shift in the management of GI conditions. The use of AI is revolutionizing how gastroenterologists diagnose and treat patients. The imaging data from endoscopies still requires a skilled clinician to perform the procedure to capture the data. Therefore, at least soon, gastroenterologists will likely use AI as an assistive tool rather than a replacement for the human eye.

By codifying expert skills in a real-time algorithm, AI automatically transfers GI pathology knowledge from experts to the gastroenterology community. This human-machine interaction will improve patient outcomes because it will augment the skills of the physician performing the procedure. In addition to its clinical advantages, AI has exciting potential as an educational tool. It can help physicians learn from their mistakes and colleagues' mistakes, thus improving patient care overall.

Integrating different stand-alone algorithms into a cohesive whole can provide more accurate diagnoses and better treatment plans for our patients. Navigation software improves our ability to visualize lesions accurately, while CADx helps us determine if further biopsy or treatment is necessary. Delineation software makes it easier for us to excise tumors completely during endoscopic procedures.

With all these stand-alone algorithms working together to create an integrated approach that benefits both doctors and patients alike, doctors can focus on other tasks, and rely on AI technology to handle lesion detection and diagnosis, allowing them more time for patient care overall. Patients also benefit from this technology as they receive timely diagnoses and high-quality, potentially life-saving treatments. All should embrace this technology.

However, one must be cautious before widespread adoption is endorsed. The following concerns must be addressed. It is imperative to question their strength and clinical validity critically. Some essential questions to ask are:

- What is the sample size of the training and validation datasets?

- Was the system trained and tested on images, postprocedural videos, or live procedures?

- Is the system capable of real-time assessment with minimal lag time?

- What improvement does this system offer, and does it have clinical benefit, in the form of decreased reaction time, improved ADR, accuracy in the characterization of abnormalities for targeted biopsies, assessment of the quality of endoscopic views, and important anatomic landmarks?

- Was the system tested against expert endoscopists in validation?

Even if we have a well-trained model, considering the ethical and legal liabilities involved if a lesion is missed, relying on AI solely will not be wise. In the end, is it the gastroenterologist, the AI algorithm developer, or the hospital that shoulders malpractice claims? Is it all of them?

CHAPTER 13

ROBOTIC SURGERY

da Vinci   **da Vinci – surgery on a grape**   **Stitching a grape back together**

The Past

Robotic surgery has a long and illustrious history, dating back to the early 1800s. The first recorded use of a robotic surgical tool was in 1806 when the French surgeon Baron Dominique Jean Larrey used a metal claw to remove a tumor from the neck of Emperor Napoleon Bonaparte. However, it was not until the late 20th century that robotic surgery began to be widely used.

The US military was the driving force for the development that would ultimately lead to robotic surgery. Realizing that hemorrhagic shock and trauma were the most frequent causes of death in combat, the military sought to provide remote expert surgical care to reduce the mortality and morbidity in the battlefield, a concept known as telepresence. In the 1980s,

SRI International, a company in Menlo Park, CA, was contracted by the US military to develop a robotic system that could allow surgeons to operate remotely on soldiers in the battlefield.[192][193]

While the military vision of telepresence never manifested, a young surgeon, Frederic Moll, discovered this technology and created a company that would ultimately become Intuitive Surgical, Inc. (ISRG). In 1997, Jacques Himpens and Guy Cardierre in Belgium performed the world's first laparoscopic cholecystectomy using a robotically-controlled instrument called "The da Vinci Surgical System".

The Present

Robotic surgery has since revolutionized surgical care and patient outcomes worldwide. Robotic surgery offers many advantages over traditional open surgery. The benefits for robotic surgery patients include smaller incisions, less pain and blood loss, less scarring, faster recovery, and shorter hospital stays than traditional surgery. In addition, robotic surgery is often less expensive than conventional open surgery.

For the surgeon, the advantages of using robotic surgery are apparent. For one thing, robots offer unparalleled precision due to their three-dimensional capabilities. This high degree of accuracy minimizes damage to surrounding tissue and results in quicker patient recoveries. Because surgeons from afar control surgical robots, they offer more dexterity than even the most skilled human hands. This allows surgeons greater flexibility when performing procedures and decreases the chances of inadvertent human mistakes, as the robots are less susceptible to fatigue and hand tremors. Hence, robotic surgery may allow surgeons to perform complex procedures that would otherwise be difficult or impossible using traditional techniques. For instance, we can program robotic surgeons to perform specific tasks with great accuracy, making them ideal for delicate procedures like brain tumor removal or cardiac valve repairs. For these reasons, robotic surgery has become the preferred choice for many surgical procedures.

Developed by ISRG, da Vinci Robot is the world's most advanced and widely used robotic surgical system. The da Vinci Robot allows surgeons to perform a wide range of complex procedures with greater precision, using a few small incisions instead of one large incision. The robot gives surgeons a 3D view of the operative field, allowing them to work more accurately and safely than ever before. For example, the robot can rotate 360 degrees around its axis, allowing surgeons to view their work from any angle. This reduces trauma to the patient's body and results in faster healing times. Since the FDA approved it in 2000, the da Vinci robot has been used for nearly 7 million surgeries worldwide.

Robotic systems are used for various surgeries, including prostatectomies, hysterectomies, coronary artery bypass graft surgery, cardiac valve repairs, and gastric bypass procedures. One study found that patients who underwent robotic prostatectomy had significantly shorter hospital stays (1.5 days vs. 2.6 days) and were less likely to require blood transfusions than those who underwent traditional open prostatectomy.[194]

The use of robotics in gastric bypass provides superior visualization, more degrees of freedom, and better ergonomics when compared to traditional surgery. This results in a quicker, less invasive, and more accurate surgical procedure for the patient. In addition, the operative time is significantly shorter with robotic surgery.[195]

A recent study showed that women undergoing hysterectomy via robotics reported less pain and shorter hospital stays than those undergoing traditional laparoscopic hysterectomies.[196] Since the introduction of robotic surgery in gynecology, the rate of cases done through this method increased from 2.5 percent to 25 percent, indicating that patients and surgeons alike find robotic surgery more valuable. This increase in popularity can be attributed to the many benefits that robotic surgery offers over traditional methods, including less pain, shorter hospital stays, and faster recoveries.[197]

Robotic-assisted cardiac surgery is also growing in popularity, as it is safer and more effective than traditional heart surgeries. A four-year study by York Hospital in Pennsylvania showed that robotic-assisted cardiac surgery increased by 600 percent, mainly because these robots allow more precision during the operation, shorter recovery time, and generally better clinical outcomes for patients.[198] In fact, the American Heart Association recently issued a statement recommending that all high-risk coronary artery bypass grafting procedures be performed using robotics whenever possible.[199]

While the development of robotic surgery has been generally led by ISRG, a company with a market capitalization of over $60 billion, newer technology companies have emerged and introduced a significant element of competition and choice to this rapidly evolving field in the past few years. Following are some of the major companies developing robots for use in surgery.

Medtronic is another major player in the robotics for surgery field. They offer the StealthStation® Robotic Surgery System, which allows surgeons to perform complex procedures through tiny incisions using miniature instruments controlled by robotic arms, treating conditions such as degenerative disc disease, spondylolisthesis, and spinal stenosis. The company's market capitalization stands at over $115 billion.

Johnson & Johnson (JNJ) offers their line of robot-assisted surgical devices through their subsidiary Ethicon, Inc. One such device is the Monarch® Platform surgery system: The first and only multispecialty, flexible robotic solution for use in both bronchoscopy and urology. JNJ's market cap clocks in at just under $350 billion.

Hansen Medical developed the Magellan robot, which is used for coronary procedures such as angioplasty and stenting.

Verb Surgical is a joint venture between Google's parent company Alphabet Inc., Johnson & Johnson, and Verily Life Sciences LLC, which focuses on developing robotics-assisted surgery technologies. (Imagine that: Google is now in the surgical robot business!)

Medrobotics Corporation has created the Flex Robotic System, a snake-like robot designed to navigate through hard-to-reach and tight spaces in the body to perform procedures such as prostatectomies and colonoscopies.

Stryker Corporation offers the Mako SmartRobotics surgery system and Smith & Nephew the NAVIO PFS system, both are designed to assist surgeons with knee replacement surgeries.

Each of these companies has developed a unique robotic platform with specific capabilities designed to improve the accuracy and safety of surgeries performed by surgeons globally.

The Future

The future of surgery is robotic! Robotic surgery is quickly becoming the standard of care for many procedures. It is here to serve and assist humans, not to replace humans. Given all these advantages, it is no surprise that robotic surgery is becoming increasingly popular in low-resource and rural areas. In fact, according to one study, nearly 60 percent of hospitals with 50 or fewer beds use robots for minimally invasive surgeries.[200] This trend will only continue as surgeons become more skilled at using this technology, and its benefits become better known.

One of the most significant benefits of robotic surgery is that it can be performed remotely. This means that surgeons can operate on patients not located near a major hospital or medical center. For example, a surgeon in a large city could perform a complex procedure on a patient living in a rural town. This would be impossible with traditional surgery in cases where a surgeon is not available to perform a complicated operation. In

2001, a transatlantic cholecystectomy was undertaken using the ZEUS system, with the operating surgeon performing the procedure in New York while the patient was physically in Strasbourg, France.[201]

Robotic surgery technology constantly evolves, and new surgery applications are continually developed. Patients will have access to more advanced surgical treatments, and their chances for a successful outcome are better than ever. Indeed, there will be boundless innovation in this field.

We could also leverage big data in surgery to rapidly help trainees and inexperienced surgeons acquire surgical knowledge and experience. With AI, we can use big data to carry the entirety of the field's knowledge, thus bringing expert surgeons' decision-making capabilities and techniques into every operating room in real-time. This would lead to technology-augmented real-time clinical decision support, which could help surgeons make better decisions during surgery, reducing surgical errors and improving patient outcomes.

Final Thoughts

While there are certainly some advantages to using robotics in place of conventional surgical techniques, it's important to note that not all procedures are suitable for robot-assisted surgery. Some operations, such as open-heart surgery or hysterectomies, still require large incisions and manual dexterity that current robots cannot replicate.

Furthermore, adverse events related to robotic surgical systems have been reported. In 2015, researchers at the University of Illinois at Urbana-Champaign, Illinois, retrospectively analyzed the performance of surgical robots over the past decade or so. Although more than 140 deaths and nearly 1400 injuries were reported, most cases were completed without incident. Interestingly, adverse outcomes were more common in complex surgical procedures, such as cardiothoracic surgery, than in general and gynecologic surgery.[202] The findings suggest that human surgeons are better equipped to perform complex surgeries while robots can handle more routine procedures.

In the future, as technology advances and robotic surgeons start working independently from human surgeons, laying the blame when things go wrong will become more complex. For instance, can a robotic surgeon be sued for malpractice? Will the surgeon overseeing the procedure be held accountable, or should the company that manufactured the robot be responsible?

For human surgeons, medical negligence has been established for quite some time. A surgeon is liable for damages if they operate negligently and cause injury to the patient. To prove that a surgeon was negligent, the patient must show that the surgeon failed to meet the standard of care in their community. There are no similar performance standards regarding artificial intelligence, and malpractice remains a legal gray area.

CHAPTER 14

PITFALLS AND LIMITATIONS

There is a lot of excitement around the potential for AI in medicine, and rightly so. Accenture Consulting has predicted that the role of artificial intelligence in medicine will grow from $600 million in 2014 to $6.6 billion in 2021.[203] However, pitfalls and limitations exist to limit its widespread use:

AI's narrow intelligence black box problem potential bias in algorithms data security and privacy systems errors cyber-attacks and ransomware new technology approval by the FDA widespread adoption

Let us consider each of these limitations.

Narrow intelligence. We can only use AI for specific tasks that are programmed into it. AI is not good at generalizing from one situation to another, an essential attribute of human intelligence. For example, if you show an AI program a picture of a cat, it will be able to find other cats in images but won't be able to identify a dog. This limitation could lead to incorrect diagnoses or treatments if the AI program isn't adequately trained on all the relevant data. This means that its usefulness is restricted and not a replacement for human intelligence. It is essential to tread carefully and remember that machines do not have logical thinking like humans. Each machine can do its narrow task, but no machine has the kind of general intelligence that can take knowledge in one domain and transfer it to another field, which is the hallmark of human intelligence.

AI also lacks human intuition. One advantage humans have over machines is our ability to use intuition and common sense when making decisions. Machines don't have this ability yet, so there is always the risk that they will make bad decisions based on faulty logic or inaccurate datasets.

Another potential pitfall with AI use in medicine, and other fields, is the **black box problem**, meaning the workings of many AI programs are opaque and complex for humans to understand. It is often difficult to understand why an algorithm makes a particular diagnosis. For example, if a black box algorithm recommends a specific cancer treatment, how can we be sure that the recommendation is correct? This is a massive issue in medicine for both physicians and patients. Unlike more-traditional software where a programmer defines the rules (e.g., a hexagon has six sides), in deep learning, the algorithm finds the rules, often without leaving an audit trail to explain its decisions. The machine renders a verdict without any accompanying evidence! This makes it difficult to determine why the software made a particular decision or how we improve it. This can also be problematic if something goes wrong with the program, and no one knows how to fix it.

For example, consider an AI tool developed to detect skin cancer. While highly accurate, no one was sure exactly which features of a mole the algorithm used to classify it as cancerous or benign. Dermatologists often use a ruler to measure potentially cancerous lesions. When slides of skin lesions were used to train the algorithm, it was found that the algorithm more often returned a positive diagnosis of cancer when a ruler was present in the submitted image.

In mission-critical applications like medical diagnosis, airlines, and security, people must feel confident in the reasoning behind the program. It is challenging to trust systems that do not explain or justify their conclusions. Neural networks are like a pile of linear algebra; connections with millions or even billions of numbers or vectors are challenging to examine and understand. It is like trying to understand what is going on inside someone's mind by slicing open their head to look at their neurons firing. We need to be mindful of this drawback of AI and use it with caution, but it shouldn't discourage us from adopting it.

In medicine, the black box problem, or how the benefit sometimes comes about by unknown means, is not unique to AI. For example, using drugs like anesthetic gases or lithium, we don't know their mechanism of action or how they do what they do. Still, we know that gases work to induce general anesthesia, and lithium treats bipolar mood disorders effectively.

Another limitation in the broad adoption of AI is the problem of data, algorithmic, and human **biases**, which can lead to misdiagnosis and potentially fatal outcomes. Let's look at a recent example in a paper by Obermeyer et al., which was published in the leading journal *Science* in 2019.[204] The researchers discovered a troubling flaw in an AI algorithm designed to help insurance companies predict preventable complications in high-risk diabetic patients, using high cost and utilization of healthcare consumption as surrogates for complicated disease. The algorithm in question was found to have a racial bias, effectively helping healthier White patients cut in line ahead of sicker Black patients for access to extra help with their chronic health needs. So, why did the algorithm fast-track access to White over Black patients? The researchers concluded that the algorithmic bias boiled down to the observation that Black patients were less likely to get the medical care they needed due to cost and lack of access. This meant that these patients were *invisible* to insurers trying to identify the high-risk patients who required interventions to prevent hospitalization or disease complications. In essence, due to a flawed line of reasoning written into the computer code, the algorithm made Black patients appear healthier than they were.

When the researchers corrected the problem and reanalyzed the data, the percentage of Black patients eligible for extra care jumped from 17.7 percent to 46.5 percent. This was an unintentional error, nonetheless unacceptable. The good news is that many of these algorithmic biases can be fixed and prevented. We must ensure that all patients are given the same level of care and treatment, regardless of race or ethnicity, and algorithms must be carefully designed to avoid violating this basic principle.

The take-home message is that AI technology is only as good as the data we feed it. Garbage in, garbage out, or bias in, bias out; failing to recognize bias in an algorithm could lead to exponentially calamitous consequences.

AI technology is also limited by the humans who design it. There appears to be a lack of diversity in the training materials for AI algorithms, which means that these algorithms have some inherent bias. It is a fact that disparate ethnic groups or residents of different regions may have unique physiologies and environmental factors that will influence the presentation of the disease. It is well-documented that minorities are underrepresented in clinical research. This raises concerns about whether these AI algorithms are genuinely impartial and unbiased. To mitigate these biases, researchers must be especially vigilant and take steps to correct them.

Another reason for algorithmic bias is the lack of diversity among the teams writing the actual code. Writing bias into the algorithm is mainly due to poorly designed questions and logical oversights. The programmers working on such software can consciously or unconsciously influence an algorithm. They can unconsciously implement values and beliefs about the world into the code while willingly leaving out some parameters that would be more representative of other populations. For example, the humans conducting the research select the slides or images used to train the machines that could exhibit unconscious bias, the tendency to make judgments without realizing it.

A Ghanaian American researcher at MIT and founder of The Algorithmic Justice League, Joy Buolamwini, reported that facial recognition software had trouble reading the faces of people with darker skin.[205] When she tested the technology on herself, she discovered the software worked better when she wore a white face mask than her actual face.

Therefore, the scientists developing the algorithms must identify the bias in the data to understand the bias in the algorithm and account for it. One way to do this is through diversity in clinical trials. When designing trials, researchers must create algorithms using data inclusive of race, gender, and socioeconomic backgrounds. Diverse groups make for better data, representing a more comprehensive range of experiences. Another way to reduce bias is through transparency. All decisions made by AI algorithms should be traceable so that their reasoning can be examined and questioned. All data used in developing AI algorithms must be made public so we can scrutinize it for potential biases.

Data security and privacy. The privacy and security of patient healthcare data are significant concerns. The large tech giants such as Google, Facebook, and Amazon appear to have access to personal information about millions of people. Many people don't understand how their data is used or why, and many companies aren't forthcoming with this information either. For instance, a data breach occurred in the UK when the Royal Free NHS Foundation Trust shared data of over 1.6 million patients with Google's DeepMind without the patients' consent.[206] The data transfer was part of a collaboration to create the healthcare app Streams, an alert, diagnosis, and detection system for acute kidney injury.

Tech companies could theoretically sell their AI-acquired healthcare data to third parties like marketers, employers, and insurers. While the Portability and Accountability Act (HIPAA) forbids healthcare providers and insurers from obtaining or disclosing patient information without consent, it does not apply to other types of businesses. As a result, there is a real danger that our most sensitive personal data will be used without our knowledge or consent for purposes we disagree with. This data can also be misused by employers or insurance companies and have profound consequences on our lives. Employers may use our data to discriminate against us in job applications, while insurance companies may use it to increase our healthcare premiums. We must be careful about who has access to our personal information and ensure that it is used only for legitimate purposes. We should demand transparency from those who collect and store our data and hold them accountable if they violate our trust. Cyber theft, ransomware, and hacking are tangible threats to our personal data. We need regulations in place that will secure and protect our privacy rights.

Another pitfall with AI is **system errors** that could have devastating consequences in medicine. The most obvious risk is that AI systems will sometimes be wrong, and that patient injury or other healthcare problems may result. I described earlier how an algorithm effectively low-balled the health needs of Black patients. Another study using data from nearly 30,000 patients in University of Michigan hospitals found that the AI algorithm used in the Epic Sepsis Model (ESM) to predict sepsis performed poorly, as it missed two-thirds of sepsis cases.[207]

Ensuring the accuracy of data will be critical for the successful implementation of AI into medicine. For example, suppose an algorithm was trained on old medical records that were not updated with current information about a patient's condition or allergies. In that case, it could lead to an incorrect diagnosis or treatment plan for that patient. Or if an AI system recommends the wrong drug for a patient, fails to notice a tumor on a radiological scan, or allocates a hospital bed to one patient over another because it predicted wrongly which patient would benefit more, patients could be injured. And if AI systems become widespread, an underlying problem in one AI system might result in injuries to thousands or millions or billions of patients versus the limited number of patients injured by any single provider's error.

Cyber-attacks and ransomware are other potential pitfalls. Malware could exploit vulnerabilities in AI systems and cause damage or loss of life. What happens if someone comes up with, let's say, a generative adversarial network algorithm to generate fake positive cancer diagnoses? These examples demonstrate that algorithmic errors can have catastrophic consequences for patients and their families. We must ensure that these errors are minimized as much as possible. One way we can do this is by ensuring that algorithms are appropriately tested and validated before they are used in the real-world and regularly updated based on new information. The AMA has proposed that AI training be incorporated as a standard component of medical education. Hospitals and other practices are also vital in ensuring proper development, implementation, and monitoring of protocols and best practices for using AI systems in medicine.

The FDA is often seen as a hurdle in new technology approvals. AI-based medical devices and algorithms must go through rigorous processes that are time – and resource-consuming. This can be considered pivotal as a barrier to introducing AI in medicine.

The FDA's approval process for AI-based medical devices includes pre-market review, post-market surveillance, and regulatory science research. To undergo pre-market review, developers must submit data on the safety and effectiveness of their device to the FDA. The agency then evaluates this data to determine if the device is safe and effective enough to be marketed in the US. If it is not approved during the pre-market review, it cannot be sold in the US market until post-market surveillance has been completed successfully. This step involves tracking how well the device performs after it has been released for use by patients. Any problems that arise must be reported back to the FDA to decide whether further action needs to be taken concerning regulating or banning the device altogether. Finally, developers must conduct regulatory science research to understand how we can safely and effectively use AI in healthcare settings.

This comprehensive approval process may seem like a hindrance to innovation; however, it exists primarily out of concern for patient safety. Developers of AI often find this process burdensome. This process can take many months, or even years, to complete. This can sometimes be a barrier to the broader implementation of AI within healthcare settings. Furthermore, when approval is granted, software upgrades and newer versions may already exist, rendering the original product obsolete. The FDA has responded to this issue by creating a program called "Pre-cert," which aims to streamline the process for developers of AI-based medical devices. This could be a significant step forward in ensuring patients have faster access to innovative AI technology in healthcare.

Finally, concerning the **widespread adoption** of AI in daily clinical practice, we are still some way off from the actual clinical deployment of these models. There are several reasons for this. Firstly, using these models requires additional technology and infrastructure that many hospitals may not yet have in place. Secondly, learning how to make an utterly digital diagnosis with an AI model takes time. Clinicians must be confident that they can trust the results before using them clinically. So, until we can seamlessly incorporate that into our current workflows, I think that will always be a barrier to the widespread adoption of AI in medicine.

Final Thoughts

Considering these potential drawbacks of AI in medicine, researchers must weigh the risks and benefits of using this innovative and potentially disruptive technology before implementing it into our daily clinical practice and workflows. We need to understand how AI will affect patients and clinicians using it. It is imperative that machine learning is paired with human-centered design to ensure a positive impact on the practice of medicine. Google Health enumerated four guiding principles for human-centered studies that have effectively developed AI technologies:[208]

1. Working with domain experts to design suitable machine learning models.

2. Performing human-computer interaction research to better understand the user and how they think.

3. Ethnographic field studies to facilitate a complete understanding of the environment in which the AI model is being deployed.

4. Collaborative design; working with the end-user experience to create better workflows.

With its many benefits, it is no wonder that AI is poised to become a staple in medicine. However, as with any new technology, some challenges come with adopting AI into medicine. Ultimately, humans decide where AI should be applied and what should be done the "old-fashioned way." If all the stakeholders strive to use AI to build the best future for patients and clinicians, this technology can change the shape of medicine. The benefits of AI outweigh its drawbacks, and we should continue to invest in this technology and explore its potential applications, as it holds great promise for the future.

CHAPTER 15

CONCLUSION

A busy young 25-year-old wife and mother of one who lives in San Francisco, Brittany also juggles a full-time career as a literary agent, matching authors with suitable publishers. For years, she has also balanced something else: stubborn and annoying headaches. A handful of different doctors had offered other diagnoses but no solution.

In October 2007, during a visit with her new family-practice physician, Brittany suggested they try and resolve the problem for good. Her doctor promptly ordered an MRI scan of her head. The day after her scan, Brittany was surprised to hear the doctor's voice on the other end of the phone. He determined the cause of her headaches and insisted she come to his office the following day. "Please tell me," Brittany pressed. "Do I have a brain tumor?"

It was not a brain tumor, but Brittany was diagnosed with a brain aneurysm. She's jerked around by the system for years, even though she has financial means. Ultimately, despite her delayed diagnosis, she reaches out to a VIP doctor in healthcare to get the best care available. It shouldn't be up to the individual with the medical illness to have to track down and plead with somebody to get the help they need. This responsibility should fall on those who are qualified and supposed to help, doctors, nurses, etc. This should not happen to anyone, regardless of their social status or wealth level.

This system is archaic, and it's time for a change. We need a healthcare system that puts the patient first, where they can easily access critical care without going through intermediaries. It's unfair and unjust that people have died or suffered because they couldn't find the right person to provide them with the necessary care at the right time. We must work together as a society, so this doesn't happen anymore. We need a healthcare system based on science, evidence, and customer service. Healthcare is an inalienable human right. Everyone should be able to access the best possible medical care without worrying about their financial status or who they know. This may be an opportunity for AI to democratize this broken system.

AI systems are increasingly used to support clinical decision-making. These systems can help identify patterns and correlations that may be difficult for humans to discern due to our limited capacity for learning and understanding. AI is currently used to facilitate early disease detection, better understand disease progression, optimize medication and treatment dosages, and uncover novel treatments.

While human learning is limited by the capacity to remember, access to knowledge sources, and lived experience, AI can synthesize information from an unlimited amount of medical information sources, allowing it to learn much faster than humans. Additionally, AI can access knowledge sources that humans cannot, making it more knowledgeable about potential treatments and interventions. For example, AI can help identify biomarkers that indicate the presence of a disease or how advanced that condition is. It can also help determine which medications will work best for each individual and what dosage would be most effective. In addition, AI may be able to find new treatments that were not successful in traditional drug trials. AI can access data from clinical trials and other real-world settings that can help inform its decisions. Additionally, AI systems can help reduce costs by automating tasks like documentation and billing. While clinicians are still necessary for many functions in the medical field, intelligent machines are becoming increasingly crucial for supporting decision-making processes.

There are many potential benefits of using AI-powered machines to support clinical decision-making:

- **Increased accuracy** – Machine learning algorithms are more accurate than humans in analyzing data. This increased accuracy could lead to better diagnosis and treatment plans for patients.

- **Faster turnaround time** – Machine learning can analyze substantial amounts of data much faster than humans, allowing results to be returned more quickly. This could improve patient outcomes by enabling clinicians better and timely access to vital information.

- **Improved efficiency** – Automated systems do not get tired or distracted like humans, leading to improved healthcare efficiency, reduced wait times, and cost savings for patients.

Despite these benefits, there are some concerns about incorporating AI into clinical decision-making processes. One worry is that reliance on machine intelligence could astray clinicians if results from algorithms are misinterpreted or incorrectly applied; if this data isn't accurate, the results could be disastrous. As machines become more involved in making decisions about patient care, questions arise about who should be responsible when something goes wrong: the clinician who inputted the information into the algorithm or the machine itself? Eventually, as with any tool used in medicine, it is vital for clinicians themselves to remain responsible for interpreting results correctly and using their judgment when making decisions about patient care. AI should never supersede human judgment in matters of life and death. Human competencies such as experience, intuition, and clinical reasoning will *always* matter.

Another concern is that increased use of AI could result in job losses among healthcare workers. As with other technological advancements throughout history, such changes typically result in new opportunities being created as well. While some risks are associated with using AI-powered machines in clinical decision-making, the potential benefits warrant further exploration.

Overall, there is no doubt that artificial intelligence has enormous potential to improve healthcare outcomes for patients worldwide. With this technology's continued development and expansion into healthcare settings, we should see even more improvements in both patient care and efficiency within the industry overall.

While I attempted to demonstrate some of the most well-known applications and some examples of what is already happening with AI in this book, there is a myriad of other applications for AI technology in healthcare that people may not be aware of, such as medical research, drug development, public health, disease surveillance, genomic sequencing, and epidemic prediction. Table 1 illustrates 29 FDA-approved AI algorithms in healthcare.

By analyzing large amounts of data, including genomic data, AI can help researchers identify new drug targets and develop new therapies faster.

In addition, AI can help automate tasks such as data entry or analysis, which can free up time for healthcare workers to focus on more critical tasks.

Public health is a critical application area for AI because it can help identify and prevent disease outbreaks before they happen. For example, AI can predict where an outbreak might occur based on data collected from social media or other sources. Nearly half of the world's population has little to no access to essential diagnostics like blood tests, pathology, and radiology.[209] This leaves them vulnerable to disease and at a disadvantage when receiving proper treatment. Without these necessary tools, people often cannot get an accurate diagnosis. By providing everyone with access to these essential tools, we can help make significant progress in global health outcomes, especially in developing countries where countless people die from preventable diseases yearly.

Epidemic prediction is another application of AI that could have a significant impact on global health. Using machine learning algorithms to analyze data about past outbreaks, we can better understand how epidemics spread and what factors contribute to them. By tracking information about diseases, including their location, prevalence, and how they are spreading, AI systems can help healthcare workers detect new outbreaks early and respond quickly. We can use this information to create models that predict when and where future outbreaks might occur. This could save lives by preventing epidemics from leaking out of control.

Genomic sequencing is another application for AI technology in healthcare that has tremendous implications for the future of medicine. With genomic sequencing, AI systems can quickly analyze large amounts of genetic data and accurately identify mutations associated with rare diseases. Sequencing genomes allows researchers to understand the role genes play in various conditions and potentially find cures for them. Additionally, genomic sequencing can help track the spread of infectious diseases.

The medical community has long heralded the promise of personalized medicine. Personalized medicine involves tailoring treatments for each patient based on their unique genetic makeup. Providing customized therapy based on a patient's genome sequencing is another application for AI in medicine. This involves using AI algorithms to analyze vast quantities of data to identify patterns we can use to predict how a particular patient will respond to a specific medication or treatment. This could allow us to provide much more individualized care for patients, increasing the likelihood that they will respond positively to treatment with minimal side effects.

Finally, a news bulletin has understandably generated concerns about the future of human clinicians and their jobs. In 2017, a Chinese medical robot named Xiaoyi passed China's medical licensing exam.[210] Xiaoyi was trained by processing dozens of medical textbooks, two million medical records, and 400,000 articles. While Xiaoyi's training was practical enough to breeze through the questions involving memorization and information recall, it didn't fare quite as well when answering questions about patient cases. So, for now, you can rest easy knowing Xiaoyi won't be replacing your job anytime soon.

Our biological brains can't process and ingest big data, and with so much data to sift through, we must start practicing medicine as a data science rather than an art. And while machines may never entirely replace clinicians, AI can help us work *smarter*. Ultimately, AI may take on more tasks that require precision and accuracy, like diagnosis or surgery. However, there are some tasks that AI cannot perform as well as humans; when it comes to empathy and the sacred doctor-patient relationship, AI falls short. Human interaction will always be an essential part of clinical care. Patients need someone to talk to and empathize with them, and they also need someone who can see the big picture and coordinate their care. Only by working alongside AI can we ensure that patients receive the best care while maintaining our unique human abilities.

One may predict that AI will never entirely take over the practice of medicine and make doctors obsolete. But clinicians who don't embrace AI technology risk being left behind as their colleagues move forward into the future of *smarter* medicine. Clinicians who don›t use artificial intelligence will eventually be replaced by those who do.

Table 15.1 Database of the 29 FDA-approved, AI/ML-based medical technologies.

#	Name of device or algorithm	Name of parent company	Short description	FDA approval number	Type of FDA approval	Mention of algorithm in announcement	Date	Medical specialty	Secondary medical specialty
1	Arterys Cardio DL	Arterys Inc.	Software analyzing cardiovascular images from MR	K163253	510(k) premarket notification	Deep learning	2016 11	Radiology	Cardiology
2	EnsoSleep	EnsoData, Inc.	Diagnosis of sleep disorders	K162627	510(k) premarket notification	Automated algorithm	2017 03	Neurology	
3	Arterys Oncology DL	Arterys Inc.	Medical diagnostic application	K173542	510(k) premarket notification	Deep learning	2017 11	Radiology	Oncology
4	Idx	IDx LLC.	Detection of diabetic retinopathy	DEN180001	de novo pathway	AI	2018 01	Ophthalmology	
5	ContaCT	Viz.AI.	Stroke detection on CT	DEN170073	de novo pathway	AI	2018 02	Radiology	Neurology

#	Name of device or algorithm	Name of parent company	Short description	FDA approval number	Type of FDA approval	Mention of algorithm in announcement	Date	Medical specialty	Secondary medical specialty
6	OsteoDetect	Imagen Technologies, Inc.	X-ray wrist fracture diagnosis	DEN180005	de novo pathway	Deep learning	2018 02	Radiology	Emergency Medicine
7	Guardian Connect System	Medtronic	Predicting blood glucose changes	P160007	PMA	AI	2018 03	Endocrinology	
8	EchoMD Automated Ejection Fraction Software	Bay Labs, Inc.	Echocardiogram analysis	K173780	510(k) premarket notification	Machine learning	2018 05	Radiology	Cardiology
9	DreaMed	DreaMed Diabetes, Ltd.	Managing Type 1 diabetes	DEN170043	de novo pathway	AI	2018 06	Endocrinology	
10	BriefCase	Aidoc Medical, Ltd.	Triage and diagnosis of time sensitive patients	K180647	510(k) premarket notification	Deep learning	2018 07	Radiology	Emergency Medicine
11	ProFound™ AI Software V2.1	iCAD, Inc.	Breast density via mammography	K191994	510(k) premarket notification	Deep learning	2018 07	Radiology	Oncology

#	Name of device or algorithm	Name of parent company	Short description	FDA approval number	Type of FDA approval	Mention of algorithm in announcement	Date	Medical specialty	Secondary medical specialty
12	SubtlePET	Subtle Medical, Inc.	Radiology image processing software	K182336	510(k) premarket notification	Deep neural network-based algorithm	2018 8	Radiology	
13	Arterys MICA	Arterys Inc.	Liver and lung cancer diagnosis on CT and MRI	K182034	510(k) premarket notification	AI	2018 09	Radiology	Oncology
14	AI-ECG Platform	Shenzhen Carewell Electronics, Ltd.	ECG analysis support	K180432	510(k) premarket notification	AI-ECG	2018 09	Cardiology	
15	Accipiolx	MaxQ-AI Ltd.	Acute intracranial hemorrhage triage algorithm	K182177	510(k) premarket notification	Artificial intelligence algorithm	2018 10	Radiology	Neurology
16	icobrain	icometrix NV	MRI brain interpretation	K181939	510(k) premarket notification	Machine learning and deep learning	2018 10	Radiology	Neurology
17	FerriSmart Analysis System	Resonance Health Analysis	Measure liver iron concentration	K182218	510(k) premarket notification	Artificial intelligence	2018 11	Internal Medicine	

#	Name of device or algorithm	Name of parent company	Short description	FDA approval number	Type of FDA approval	Mention of algorithm in announcement	Date	Medical specialty	Secondary medical specialty
		Service Pty Ltd.							
18	cmTriage	CureMetrix, Inc.	Mammogram workflow	K183285	510(k) premarket notification	Artificial intelligence algorithm	2019 03	Radiology	Oncology
19	Deep Learning Image Reconstruction	GE Medical Systems, LLC.	CT image reconstruction	K183202	510(k) premarket notification	Deep learning	2019 04	Radiology	
20	HealthPNX	Zebra Medical Vision Ltd.	Chest X-Ray assessment pneumothorax	K190362	510(k) premarket notification	Artificial intelligence	2019 05	Radiology	Emergency Medicine
21	Advanced Intelligent Clear-IQ Engine (AiCE)	Canon Medical Systems Corporation	Noise reduction algorithm	K183046	510(k) premarket notification	Deep Convolutional Neural Network	2019 06	Radiology	
22	SubtleMR	Subtle Medical, Inc.	Radiology image processing software	K191688	510(k) premarket notification	Convolutional neural network	2019 7	Radiology	

#	Name of device or algorithm	Name of parent company	Short description	FDA approval number	Type of FDA approval	Mention of algorithm in announcement	Date	Medical specialty	Secondary medical specialty
23	AI-Rad Companion (Pulmonary)	Siemens Medical Solutions USA, Inc.	CT image reconstruction - pulmonary	K183271	510(k) premarket notification	Deep learning	2019 07	Radiology	
24	Critical Care Suite	GE Medical Systems, LLC.	Chest X-Ray assessment pneumothorax	K183182	510(k) premarket notification	Artificial intelligence algorithms	2019 08	Radiology	Emergency Medicine
25	AI-Rad Companion (Cardiovascular)	Siemens Medical Solutions USA, Inc.	CT image reconstruction - cardiovascular	K183268	510(k) premarket notification	Deep learning	2019 09	Radiology	
26	EchoGo Core	Ultromics Ltd.	Quantification and reporting of results of cardiovascular function	K191171	510(k) premarket notification	Machine learning-based algorithms	2019 11	Cardiology	Radiology
27	Transpara TM	Screenpoint Medical B.V.	Mammogram workflow	K192287	510(k) premarket notification	Machine learning components	2019 12	Radiology	Oncology

#	Name of device or algorithm	Name of parent company	Short description	FDA approval number	Type of FDA approval	Mention of algorithm in announcement	Date	Medical specialty	Secondary medical specialty
28	QuantX	Quantitative Insights, Inc.	Radiological software for lesions suspicious for cancer	DEN170022	de novo pathway	Artificial intelligence algorithm	2020 01	Radiology	Oncology
29	Eko Analysis Software	Eko Devices Inc.	Cardiac Monitor	K192004	510(k) premarket notification	Artificial neural network	2020 01	Cardiology	

From Benjamens S, Dhunnoo P, Meskó B. The state of artificial intelligence-based FDA-approved medical devices and algorithms: An online database. NPJ Digit Med. 2020;3:118. Published 2020 Sep 11. doi:10.1038/s41746-020-00324-0. Open Access Creative Commons CC BY 4.0 license https://creativecommons.org/licenses/by/4.0/

ACKNOWLEDGMENT

I wish to express my gratitude to my colleagues Felicia Faulkner for her help in creating this book's title and to Henry Artime for helping me with the graphic design.

ENDNOTES

1 Nilsson Nils J. Artificial Intelligence: A New Synthesis. Ukraine, Elsevier Science, 1998.

2 Voiland A. How Algorithm Got Its Name. Earth Observatory, NASA. August 20, 2017. Accessed May 2, 2022. https://earthobservatory.nasa.gov/images/91544/how-algorithm-got-its-name

3 Turing AM. On Computable Numbers, with an Application to the Entscheidungsproblem. A Correction. Proceedings of the London Mathematical Society. 1938;2.43(6):544–6.

4 What Consumers Really Think About AI. Pega. Accessed May 2, 2022. https://www1.pega.com/system/files/resources/2017-11/what-con-sumers-really-think-of-ai-infographic.pdf

5 Cann O. Machines Will Do More Tasks Than Humans by 2025 but Robot Revolution Will Still Create 58 Million Net New Jobs in Next Five Years. September 17, 2018. Accessed May 2, 2022. https://www.weforum.org/press/2018/09/machines-will-do-more-tasks-than-hu-mans-by-2025-but-robot-revolution-will-still-create-58-million-net-new-jobs-in-next-five-years/

6 The Algorithm Will See You Now: How AI's Healthcare Potential Out-weighs Its Risk. The Doctors Company. October 2019. Accessed May 2, 2022. https://www.thedoctors.com/articles/the-algorithm-will-see-you-now-how-ais-healthcare-potential-outweighs-its-risk/

7 Yang J. U.S. National Health Expenditure as Percent of GDP From 1960 to 2020. Statista. December 2021. Accessed May 2, 2022. https://www.statista.com/statistics/184968/us-health-expenditure-as-percent-of-gdp-since-1960/

8 McGlynn EA, Asch SM, Adams J, et al. The quality of health care deliv-ered to adults in the United States. N Engl J Med. 2003;348(26):2635-2645. doi:10.1056/NEJMsa022615

9 Emanuel EJ. The cost-coverage trade-off: "It's health care costs, stupid". JAMA. 2008;299(8):947-949. doi:10.1001/jama.299.8.947

10 Papanicolas I, Woskie LR, Jha AK. Health Care Spending in the

United States and Other High-Income Countries [published correction appears in JAMA. 2018 May 1;319(17):1824]. JAMA. 2018;319(10):1024-1039. doi:10.1001/jama.2018.1150

11 Kurani N, Wager E. How does the quality of the U.S. health system compare to other countries? Peterson-KFF Health System Tracker. September 30, 2021. Accessed May 2, 2022. https://www.healthsystemtracker.org/chart-collection/quality-u-s-healthcare-system-compare-countries/

12 Ross J. Diagnostic Error in General Surgery: Cognitive Bias and Systems Issues in Medical Malpractice Claims (Abstract). The Doctors Company. October 2021. Accessed May 2, 2022. https://www.thedoctors.com/articles/diagnostic-error-in-general-surgery-cognitive-bias-and-systems-issues-in-medical-malpractice-claims-abstract/

13 Adhikari NKJ. Patient safety without borders: measuring the global burden of adverse events. BMJ Quality & Safety 2013;22:798-801.

14 Desjardins J. How Much Data Is Generated Each Day? World Economic Forum. April 17, 2019. Accessed May 2, 2022. https://www.weforum.org/agenda/2019/04/how-much-data-is-generated-each-day-cf4bddf29f/

15 Obermeyer Z, Cohn B, Wilson M, Jena AB, Cutler DM. Early death after discharge from emergency departments: analysis of national US insurance claims data. BMJ 2017;356:j239 doi:10.1136/bmj.j239

16 Harari YN. Homo Deus: A History of Tomorrow. HarperCollins. 2015.

17 Topol EJ. Deep Medicine: How Artificial Intelligence Can Make Healthcare Human Again. United States: Basic Books. 2019

18 Topol EJ. Deep Medicine: How Artificial Intelligence Can Make Healthcare Human Again. United States: Basic Books. 2019

19 Fox R. Pharmacists Commit More Than Two Million Prescription Errors Every Year. Sommers Schwartz. December 2018. Accessed May 2, 2022. https://www.sommerspc.com/blog/2018/12/pharmacists-commit-more-than-two-million-prescription-errors-every-year/

20 Tenopir C, King DW, Clarke MT, Na K, Zhou X. Journal reading patterns and preferences of pediatricians. J Med Libr Assoc. 2007;95(1):56-63.

21 Fiorini N, Lipman DJ, Lu Z. Towards PubMed 2.0. Elife.

2017;6:e28801. Published 2017 Oct 30. doi:10.7554/eLife.28801

22 Patel NM, Michelini VV, Snell JM, Balu S, et al. Enhancing Next-Generation Sequencing-Guided Cancer Care Through Cognitive Computing. Oncologist. 2018 Feb;23(2):179-185.

23 Lee K-F. AI Superpowers: China, Silicon Valley, and the New World Order. Houghton Mifflin Harcourt. New York, New York. 2018.

24 Robertson SL, Robinson MD, Reid A. Electronic Health Record Effects on Work-Life Balance and Burnout Within the I3 Population Collaborative. J Grad Med Educ. 2017;9(4):479-484. doi:10.4300/JGME-D-16-00123.1

25 Hsiao CJ, Jha AK, King J, Patel V, Furukawa MF, Mostashari F. Office-based physicians are responding to incentives and assistance by adopting and using electronic health records. Health Aff (Millwood). 2013;32(8):1470-1477. doi:10.1377/hlthaff.2013.0323

26 Foster C. University of New Mexico Studies Physician Burnout Related to Electronic Records. The University of New Mexico Health Sciences Newsroom. September 23, 2019. Accessed May 2, 2022. https://hsc.unm.edu/news/news/university-of-new-mexico-studies-physician-burnout-related-to-electronic-records.html

27 Topol EJ. Deep Medicine: How Artificial Intelligence Can Make Healthcare Human Again. United States: Basic Books. 2019

28 Sinsky C, Colligan L, Li L, et al. Allocation of Physician Time in Ambulatory Practice: A Time and Motion Study in 4 Specialties. Ann Intern Med. 2016;165(11):753-760. doi:10.7326/M16-0961

29 Farmer B. When Doctors Struggle with Suicide, Their Profession Often Fails Them. NPR. July 31, 2018. Accessed May 2, 2022. https://www.npr.org/sections/health-shots/2018/07/31/634217947/to-prevent-doctor-suicides-medical-industry-rethinks-how-doctors-work

30 Wang MD, Khanna R, Najafi N. Characterizing the Source of Text in Electronic Health Record Progress Notes. JAMA Intern Med. 2017;177(8):1212-1213. doi:10.1001/jamainternmed.2017.1548

31 Using an AI Assistant to Reduce Documentation Burden in Family Medicine. Innovation Labs Report: Evaluating the Suki Assistant. American Academy of Family Physicians. November 2021. Accessed May 2, 2022. https://www.aafp.org/dam/AAFP/documents/practice_management/innovation_lab/report-suki-assistant-documenta-

tion-burden.pdf

32 Meskó B. Director of The Medical F There Is No Precision Medicine Without Artificial Intelligence. LinkedIn. October 23, 2017. Accessed May 2, 2022. https://www.linkedin.com/pulse/precision-medi-cine-without-artificial-intelligence-mesk%C3%B3-md-phd/

33 Wright AA, Katz IT. Beyond Burnout – Redesigning Care to Restore Meaning and Sanity for Physicians. N Engl J Med. 2018;378(4):309-311. doi:10.1056/NEJMp1716845

34 Hoyer C, Szabo K. Pitfalls in the Diagnosis of Posterior Circulation Stroke in the Emergency Setting. Front Neurol. 2021;12:682827. Published 2021 Jul 14. doi:10.3389/fneur.2021.682827

35 Brown J. Posterior Stroke, HiNTS exam. emDocs. January 22, 2015. Accessed May 3, 2022. http://www.emdocs.net/posteri-or-stroke-hints-exam/

36 Garcia TC, Bernstein AB, Bush MA. Emergency department visitors and visits: Who used the emergency room in 2007. NCHS Data Brief 2010;38:1-8. http://www.cdc.gov/nchs/data/databriefs/db38.pdf

37 Obermeyer Z, Cohn B, Wilson M, Jena AB, Cutler DM. Early death after discharge from emergency departments: analysis of national US insurance claims data. BMJ 2017;356:j239 doi:10.1136/bmj.j239

38 Meyer AN, Longhurst CA, Singh H. Crowdsourcing Diagnosis for Patients With Undiagnosed Illnesses: An Evaluation of CrowdMed. J Med Internet Res. 2016;18(1):e12. Published 2016 Jan 14. doi:10.2196/jmir.4887

39 Muse ED, Godino JG, Netting JF, Alexander JF, Moran HJ, Topol EJ. From second to hundredth opinion in medicine: A global consultation platform for physicians. NPJ Digit Med. 2018;1:55. Published 2018 Oct 9. doi:10.1038/s41746-018-0064-y

40 RARE DISEASE DAY® WITH NORD. National Organization for Rare Disorders, Inc. 2019. Accessed May 3, 2022. https://rarediseases.org/wp-content/uploads/2019/01/RDD-FAQ-2019.pdf

41 Topol EJ. Deep Medicine: How Artificial Intelligence Can Make Healthcare Human Again. United States: Basic Books. 2019

42 Bayes' Theorem. Stanford Encyclopedia of Philosophy. Updated September 30, 200. Accessed May 3, 2022. https://plato.stanford.edu/

entries/bayes-theorem/

43 Sanders L. Why we need medical diagnosis detectives. Youtube. Jul 15, 2020. Accessed May 3, 2022. https://www.youtube.com/ watch?v=qHlZWtxyAYc

44 Singh H, Meyer AN, Thomas EJ. The frequency of diagnostic errors in outpatient care: estimations from three large observational studies involving US adult populations. BMJ Qual Saf. 2014;23(9):727-731. doi:10.1136/bmjqs-2013-002627

45 National Academies of Sciences, Engineering, and Medicine. Improving Diagnosis in Health Care. Washington, DC: The National Academies Press. 2015.

46 Van Such M, Lohr R, Beckman T, Naessens JM. Extent of diagnostic agreement among medical referrals. J Eval Clin Pract. 2017;23(4):870-874. doi:10.1111/jep.12747

47 Schiff GD, Hasan O, Kim S, et al. Diagnostic error in medicine: analysis of 583 physician-reported errors. Arch Intern Med. 2009;169(20):1881-1887. doi:10.1001/archinternmed.2009.333

48 Tehrani ASS, Lee HW, Mathews SC, et al. 25-Year summary of US malpractice claims for diagnostic errors 1986-2010: an analysis from the National Practitioner Data Bank. BMJ Qual Saf. 2013;22(8):672-680. doi:10.1136/bmjqs-2012-001550.

49 Exponential Medicine. Exponential Growth of Bad Medicine with Isaac Kohane. Youtube. Oct 15, 2015. Accessed May 3, 2022. https://youtu.be/pi1O4_FskZM

50 Moore LG. Escaping the tyranny of the urgent by delivering planned care. Fam Pract Manag. 2006;13(5):37-40.

51 Reis BY, Kohane IS, Mandl KD. Longitudinal histories as predictors of future diagnoses of domestic abuse: Modelling study BMJ 2009; 339 :b3677 doi:10.1136/bmj.b3677

52 Barak-Corren Y, Castro VM, Javitt S, et al. Predicting Suicidal Behavior From Longitudinal Electronic Health Records. Am J Psychiatry. 2017;174(2):154-162. doi:10.1176/appi.ajp.2016.16010077

53 Manrai AK, Bhatia G, Strymish J, Kohane IS, Jain SH. Medicine's Uncomfortable Relationship With Math: Calculating Positive Predictive Value. JAMA Intern Med. 2014;174(6):991–993. doi:10.1001/jamaint-

ernmed.2014.1059

54 Casscells W, Schoenberger A, Graboys TB. Interpretation by physicians of clinical laboratory results. N Engl J Med. 1978;299(18):999-1001.

55 Song Z, Kannan S, Gambrel RJ, et al. Physician Practice Pattern Variations in Common Clinical Scenarios Within 5 US Metropolitan Areas. JAMA Health Forum. 2022;3(1):e214698. doi:10.1001/jamahealthforum.2021.4698

56 Liang H, Tsui BY, Ni H, et al. Evaluation and accurate diagnoses of pediatric diseases using artificial intelligence. Nat Med. 2019 Mar;25(3):433-438.

57 Reis BY, Kohane IS, Mandl KD. Longitudinal histories as predictors of future diagnoses of domestic abuse: Modelling study BMJ 2009; 339 :b3677 doi:10.1136/bmj.b3677

58 Schwartz WB. Medicine and the computer. The promise and problems of change. N Engl J Med. 1970 Dec 3;283(23):1257-64.

59 Muse ED, Godino JG, Netting JF, Alexander JF, Moran HJ, Topol EJ. From second to hundredth opinion in medicine: A global consultation platform for physicians. NPJ Digit Med. 2018;1:55. Published 2018 Oct 9. doi:10.1038/s41746-018-0064-y

60 Topol EJ. Deep Medicine: How Artificial Intelligence Can Make Healthcare Human Again. United States: Basic Books. 2019

61 Robboy SJ, Weintraub S, Horvath AE, et al. Pathologist workforce in the United States: I. Development of a predictive model to examine factors influencing supply. Arch Pathol Lab Med. 2013;137(12):1723-1732. doi:10.5858/arpa.2013-0200-OA

62 Elmore JG, Barnhill RL, Elder DE, et al. Pathologists' diagnosis of invasive melanoma and melanocytic proliferations: observer accuracy and reproducibility study [published correction appears in BMJ. 2017 Aug 8;358:j3798]. BMJ. 2017;357:j2813. Published 2017 Jun 28. doi:10.1136/bmj.j2813

63 Beck AH, Sangoi AR, Leung S, et al. Systematic analysis of breast cancer morphology uncovers stromal features associated with survival. Sci Transl Med. 2011;3(108):108ra113. doi:10.1126/scitranslmed.3002564

64 Bulten W, Pinckaers H, van Boven H, et al. Automated deep-learning

system for Gleason grading of prostate cancer using biopsies: a diagnostic study. Lancet Oncol. 2020;21(2):233-241. doi:10.1016/S1470-2045(19)30739-9

65 FDA Authorizes Software that Can Help Identify Prostate Cancer. U.S. Food & Drug Administration. September 21, 2021. Accessed May 4, 2022. https://www.fda.gov/news-events/press-announcements/fda-authorizes-software-can-help-identify-prostate-cancer

66 Raciti P, Sue J, Ceballos R, et al. Novel artificial intelligence system increases the detection of prostate cancer in whole slide images of core needle biopsies. Mod Pathol. 2020;33(10):2058-2066. doi:10.1038/s41379-020-0551-y

67 Sahasrabuddhe VV, Parham GP, Mwanahamuntu MH, Vermund SH. Cervical cancer prevention in low – and middle-income countries: Feasible, affordable, essential. Cancer Prev Res (Phila). 2012;5(1):11-17. doi:10.1158/1940-6207.CAPR-11-0540

68 NIH/National Cancer Institute. AI approach outperformed human experts in identifying cervical precancer: Algorithm could revolutionize cervical cancer screening, especially in low-resource settings. ScienceDaily. January 10, 2019. Retrieved April 23, 2022 from www.sciencedaily.com/releases/2019/01/190110164701.htm

69 Lu MY, Chen TY, Williamson DFK, et al. AI-based pathology predicts origins for cancers of unknown primary. Nature. 2021;594(7861):106-110. doi:10.1038/s41586-021-03512-4

70 Topol EJ. Deep Medicine: How Artificial Intelligence Can Make Healthcare Human Again. United States: Basic Books. 2019.

71 Imagine Your World with Watson. IBM Watson Health. 2016. Accessed May 3, 2022. https://www.ibm.com/blogs/watson-health/wp-content/uploads/2016/12/WHI-Overview-Executive-Brief.pdf

72 Jha S. Commentary: Will Computers Replace Radiologists? Medscape. May 12, 2016. Accessed May 3, 2022. https://www.medscape.com/viewarticle/863127

73 Initiative Reduce Unnecessary Radiation Exposure Medical Imaging: Appropriate Use. U.S. Food & Drug Administration. June 14, 2019. Accessed May 3, 2022. https://www.fda.gov/radiation-emitting-products/initiative-reduce-unnecessary-radiation-exposure-medical-imaging/appropriate-use

74 Smith M, Saunders R, Stuckhardt L, McGinnis JM, Committee on the Learning Health Care System in America; Institute of Medicine, eds. Best Care at Lower Cost: The Path to Continuously Learning Health Care in America. Washington (DC): National Academies Press (US); May 10, 2013.

75 Jonas DE, Reuland DS, Reddy SM, et al. Screening for Lung Cancer With Low-Dose Computed Tomography: Updated Evidence Report and Systematic Review for the US Preventive Services Task Force. JAMA. 2021;325(10):971–987

76 Hubbard RA, Kerlikowske K, Flowers CI, Yankaskas BC, Zhu W, Miglioretti DL. Cumulative probability of false-positive recall or biopsy recommendation after 10 years of screening mammography: a cohort study [published correction appears in Ann Intern Med. 2014 May 6;160(9):658]. Ann Intern Med. 2011;155(8):481-492. doi:10.7326/0003-4819-155-8-201110180-00004

77 Bruno MA, Walker EA, Abujudeh HH. Understanding and confronting our mistakes: the epidemiology of error in radiology and strategies for error reduction. Radiographics. 2015;35:1668–1676

78 Berlin L, Berlin JW. Malpractice and radiologists in Cook County, IL: Trends in 20 years of litigation. Am J Roent 1995;165:781-788.

79 Limitations of Mammograms. American Cancer Society. Updated January 14, 2022. Accessed May 3, 2022. https://www.cancer.org/cancer/breast-cancer/screening-tests-and-early-detection/mammograms/limitations-of-mammograms.html

80 McKinney SM, Sieniek M, Godbole V, et al. International evaluation of an AI system for breast cancer screening [published correction appears in Nature. 2020 Oct;586(7829):E19]. Nature. 2020;577(7788):89-94. doi:10.1038/s41586-019-1799-6

81 Yala A, Mikhael PG, Strand F, et al. Toward robust mammography-based models for breast cancer risk. Sci Transl Med. 2021;13(578):eaba4373. doi:10.1126/scitranslmed.aba4373

82 Knight W. These Doctors Are Using AI to Screen for Breast Cancer. Wired. January 27, 2021. Accessed May 3, 2022. https://www.wired.com/story/doctors-using-ai-screen-breast-cancer/

83 Rosman DA, Nshizirungu JJ, Rudakemwa E, et al. Imaging in land of 1000 hills: Rwanda radiology country report. J Glob Radiol.

2015;1:1004. doi:10.7191/jgr.2015.1004

84 Risk of Dying from Cancer Continues to Drop at an Accelerated Pace. American Cancer Society. January 12, 2022. Accessed May 3, 2022. https://www.cancer.org/latest-news/facts-and-figures-2022.html

85 Jonas DE, Reuland DS, Reddy SM, et al. Screening for Lung Cancer With Low-Dose Computed Tomography: Updated Evidence Report and Systematic Review for the US Preventive Services Task Force. JAMA. 2021;325(10):971–987

86 Ardila D, Kiraly AP, Bharadwaj S, et al. End-to-end lung cancer screening with three-dimensional deep learning on low-dose chest computed tomography [published correction appears in Nat Med. 2019 Aug;25(8):1319]. Nat Med. 2019;25(6):954-961. doi:10.1038/s41591-019-0447-x

87 Artificial Intelligence May Help Diagnose Tuberculosis in Remote Areas. Jefferson University Hospitals. April 24, 2017. Accessed May 3, 2022. https://hospitals.jefferson.edu/news/2017/04/artificial-intelligence-may-help-diagnose-tuberculosis.html

88 Lakhani P, Sundaram B. Deep Learning at Chest Radiography: Automated Classification of Pulmonary Tuberculosis by Using Convolutional Neural Networks. Radiology. 2017;284(2):574-582. doi:10.1148/radiol.2017162326

89 Trebeschi S, Drago SG, Birkbak NJ, et al. Predicting response to cancer immunotherapy using noninvasive radiomic biomarkers. Ann Oncol. 2019;30(6):998-1004. doi:10.1093/annonc/mdz108

90 Wehbe RM, Sheng J, Dutta S, et al. DeepCOVID-XR: An Artificial Intelligence Algorithm to Detect COVID-19 on Chest Radiographs Trained and Tested on a Large U.S. Clinical Data Set. Radiology. 2021;299(1):E167-E176. doi:10.1148/radiol.2020203511

91 Lee CI, Elmore JG. Artificial Intelligence for Breast Cancer Imaging: The New Frontier? J Natl Cancer Inst. 2019;111(9):875-876. doi:10.1093/jnci/djy223

92 Topol EJ. Deep Medicine: How Artificial Intelligence Can Make Healthcare Human Again. United States: Basic Books. 2019

93 The Future of Radiology and Artificial Intelligence. The Medical Futurist. June 29, 2017. Accessed May 3, 2022. https://medicalfuturist.com/the-future-of-radiology-and-ai/

94 Davenport TH, Keith J. Dreyer KJ. AI Will Change Radiology, but It Won't Replace Radiologists. Harvard Business Review. March 27, 2018. Accessed May 3, 2022. https://hbr.org/2018/03/ai-will-change-radiology-but-it-wont-replace-radiologists

95 Writing Group Members, Lloyd-Jones D, Adams RJ, et al. Heart disease and stroke statistics—2010 update: A report from the American Heart Association [published correction appears in Circulation. 2010 Mar 30;121(12):e260.

96 Attia ZI, Kapa S, Lopez-Jimenez F, et al. Screening for cardiac contractile dysfunction using an artificial intelligence-enabled electrocardiogram. Nat Med. 2019;25(1):70-74. doi:10.1038/s41591-018-0240-2

97 Mayo Clinic. Artificial Intelligence in Cardiology: A Futuristic View of A.I. in Cardiology. Youtube. August 8, 2019. Accessed May 4, 2022. https://www.youtube.com/watch?v=ydB3GhmWDFc

98 AliveCor Receives First FDA Clearance to Detect a Serious Heart Condition in an ECG on a Mobile Device. AliveCor. August 21, 2014. Accessed May 4, 2022. https://www.alivecor.com/press/press_release/alivecor-receives-first-fda-clearance-to-detect-a-serious-heart-condition-in-an-ecg-on-a-mobile-device/

99 FDA Clears First Medical Device Accessory for Apple Watch®. AliveCor. November 30, 2017. Accessed May 4, 2022. https://www.alivecor.com/press/press_release/fda-clears-first-medical-device-for-apple-watch/

100 Cleveland Clinic Study Affirms Accurate Detection of Atrial Fibrillation by KardiaBand for Apple Watch. AliveCor. March 12, 2018. Accessed May 4, 2022. https://www.alivecor.com/press/press_release/cleveland-clinic-study-affirms-accurate-detection-of-atrial-fibrillation/

101 Malloy T. Mayo Clinic research yields breakthrough in mobile determination of QT prolongation. Mayo Clinic. February 1, 2021. Accessed May 4, 2022. https://newsnetwork.mayoclinic.org/discussion/mayo-clinic-research-yields-breakthrough-in-mobile-determination-of-qt-prolongation/

102 Clinical Research: 150 Peer-Reviewed Articles. AliveCor. Accessed May 4, 2022. https://www.alivecor.com/research/

103 Most Innovative Companies of 2018. Sector: Artificial Intelligence. Fast Company & Inc. Accessed May 4, 2022. https://www.fastcompany.

com/most-innovative-companies/2018/sectors/artificial-intelligence

104 Khurshid S, Friedman S, Reeder C, et al. ECG-Based Deep Learning and Clinical Risk Factors to Predict Atrial Fibrillation. Circulation. 2022;145(2):122-133. doi:10.1161/CIRCULATIONAHA.121.057480

105 HospiMedica International staff writers. AI-Based Method Predicts Atrial Fibrillation Risk Based on ECG Results. HospiMedica International. November 24, 2021. Accessed May 4, 2022. https://www. hospimedica.com/patient-care/articles/294790675/ai-based-method-predicts-atrial-fibrillation-risk-based-on-ecg-results.html

106 US Preventive Services Task Force, Curry SJ, Krist AH, et al. Risk Assessment for Cardiovascular Disease With Nontraditional Risk Factors: US Preventive Services Task Force Recommendation Statement. JAMA. 2018;320(3):272-280. doi:10.1001/jama.2018.8359

107 Eng D, Chute C, Khandwala N, et al. Automated coronary calcium scoring using deep learning with multicenter external validation. NPJ Digit Med. 2021;4(1):88. Published 2021 Jun 1. doi:10.1038/s41746-021-00460-1

108 Rogers AJ, Selvalingam A, Alhusseini MI, et al. Machine Learned Cellular Phenotypes in Cardiomyopathy Predict Sudden Death. Circ Res. 2021;128(2):172-184. doi:10.1161/CIRCRESAHA.120.317345

109 Schwab K, Nguyen D, Ungab G, et al. Artificial intelligence MacHIne learning for the detection and treatment of atrial fibrillation guidelines in the emergency department setting (AIM HIGHER): *J Am Coll Emerg Physicians Open.* 2021;2(4):e12534. Published 2021 Aug 9. doi:10.1002/emp2.12534

110 Sardar P, Abbott JD, Kundu A, Aronow HD, Granada JF, Giri J. Impact of Artificial Intelligence on Interventional Cardiology: From Decision-Making Aid to Advanced Interventional Procedure Assistance [published correction appears in JACC Cardiovasc Interv. 2019 Aug 26;12(16):1634]. JACC Cardiovasc Interv. 2019;12(14):1293-1303. doi:10.1016/j.jcin.2019.04.048

111 Stewart J, Sprivulis P, Dwivedi G. Artificial intelligence and machine learning in emergency medicine. Emerg Med Australas. 2018;30(6):870–4.

112 Syeda-Mahmood T, Walach E, Beymer D, et al. Medical sieve. A cognitive assistant for radiologists and cardiologists. Proc SPIE – Prog

Biomed Opt Imaging [Internet]. 2016;9785

113 Skin Cancer. American Academy of Dermatology Assocation. Last updated April 22, 2022. Accessed May 5, 2022. https://www.aad.org/media/stats-skin-cancer

114 Hu J, McKoy K, Papier A, et al. Dermatology and HIV/AIDS in Africa. J Glob Infect Dis. 2011;3(3):275-280. doi:10.4103/0974-777X.83535

115 Finley CR, Chan DS, Garrison S, Korownyk C, Kolber MR, Campbell S, Eurich DT, Lindblad AJ, Vandermeer B, Allan GM. What are the most common conditions in primary care? Systematic review. Can Fam Physician. 2018 Nov;64(11):832-840.

116 Onsoi W, Chaiyarit J, Techasatian L. Common misdiagnoses and prevalence of dermatological disorders at a pediatric tertiary care center. J Int Med Res. 2020;48(2):300060519873490. doi:10.1177/0300060519873490

117 Esteva A, Kuprel B, Novoa RA, et al. Corrigendum: Dermatologist-level classification of skin cancer with deep neural networks. Nature. 2017;546(7660):686. doi:10.1038/nature22985

118 Haenssle HA, Fink C, Schneiderbauer R, et al. Man against machine: diagnostic performance of a deep learning convolutional neural network for dermoscopic melanoma recognition in comparison to 58 dermatologists. Ann Oncol. 2018;29(8):1836-1842. doi:10.1093/annonc/mdy166

119 Liu Y, Jain A, Eng C, et al. A deep learning system for differential diagnosis of skin diseases. Nat Med 2020;26:900–908 (2020). Doi:10.1038/s41591-020-0842-3

120 Jain A, Way D, Gupta V, et al. Development and Assessment of an Artificial Intelligence–Based Tool for Skin Condition Diagnosis by Primary Care Physicians and Nurse Practitioners in Teledermatology Practices. JAMA Netw Open. 2021;4(4):e217249. doi:10.1001/jamanetworkopen.2021.7249

121 Bui P, Liu Y. Using AI to help find answers to common skin conditions. Google Health News. May 18, 2021. Accessed May 3, 2022. https://blog.google/technology/health/ai-dermatology-preview-io-2021/

122 3Derm announces two FDA Breakthrough Device designations for autonomous skin cancer AI. PRNewsire. January 07, 2020. Accessed

May 5, 2022. https://www.prnewswire.com/news-releases/3derm-an-nounces-two-fda-breakthrough-device-designations-for-autono-mous-skin-cancer-ai-300982072.html

123 Digital Diagnostics, formerly IDx, Expands Global Impact of Healthcare Autonomous AI with Acquisition of 3Derm Systems, Inc. Digital Diagnostics Press Release. August 19, 2020. Accessed May 5, 2022. https://www.digitaldiagnostics.com/newsroom/digital-diag-nostics-formerly-idx-expands-global-impact-of-healthcare-autono-mous-ai-with-acquisition-of-3derm-systems-inc/

124 Gomolin A, Netchiporouk E, Gniadecki R, Litvinov IV. Artificial Intelligence Applications in Dermatology: Where Do We Stand? Front Med (Lausanne). 2020;7:100. Published 2020 Mar 31. doi:10.3389/fmed.2020.00100

125 Our New Approach to a Challenging Skin Cancer Statistic. The Skin Cancer Foundation. April 1, 2021. Accessed May 5, 2022.

126 Spyridonos P, Gaitanis G, Likas A, Bassukas ID. Automatic discrim-ination of actinic keratoses from clinical photographs. Comput Biol Med. 2017;88:50–9

127 Manohar DD, Maity M, Mungle T, et al. Fuzzy spectral clustering for automated delineation of chronic wound region using digital images. Comput Biol Med. 2017;89:551-560. doi:10.1016/j.comp-biomed.2017.04.004

128 Mukherjee R, Manohar DD, Das DK, Achar A, Mitra A, Chakraborty C. Automated tissue classification framework for reproducible chronic wound assessment. Biomed Res Int. 2014;2014:851582. doi:10.1155/2014/851582

129 Alderden J, Pepper GA, Wilson A, et al. Predicting Pressure Injury in Critical Care Patients: A Machine-Learning Model. Am J Crit Care. 2018;27(6):461-468. doi:10.4037/ajcc2018525

130 Shrivastava VK, Londhe ND, Sonawane RS, Suri JS. A novel and robust Bayesian approach for segmentation of psoriasis lesions and its risk stratification. Comp Methods Programs Biomed. (2017) 150:9–22. doi: 10.1016/j.cmpb.2017.07.011

131 Wei C, Adusumilli N, Friedman A, Patel V. Perceptions of Artifi-cial Intelligence Integration into Dermatology Clinical Practice: A Cross-Sectional Survey Study. J Drugs Dermatol. 2022;21(2):135-140.

doi:10.36849/jdd.6398

132 American Diabetes Association. Introduction: Standards of Medical Care in Diabetes—2022. Diabetes Care 1 January 2022;45(Supp1):S1–S2. doi.org/10.2337/dc22-Sint

133 LeBrun N. 7 Things to Know About the Ophthalmologist Shortage. Healthgrades. Updated on December 16, 2021. Accessed May 5, 2022. https://www.healthgrades.com/pro/7-things-to-know-about-the-ophthalmologist-shortage

134 Young A. Supply and demand: Navigating the future of ophthalmology. Healio Ocular Surgery News. July 10, 2021. Accessed May 5, 2022. https://www.healio.com/news/ophthalmology/20210707/supply-and-demand-navigating-the-future-of-ophthalmology

135 Feng PW, Ahluwalia A, Feng H, Adelman RA. National Trends in the United States Eye Care Workforce from 1995 to 2017. Am J Ophthalmol. 2020;218:128-135. doi:10.1016/j.ajo.2020.05.018

136 Gulshan V, Peng L, Coram M, et al. Development and Validation of a Deep Learning Algorithm for Detection of Diabetic Retinopathy in Retinal Fundus Photographs. JAMA. 2016;316(22):2402–2410. doi:10.1001/jama.2016.17216

137 Poplin R, Varadarajan AV, Blumer K, et al. Prediction of cardiovascular risk factors from retinal fundus photographs via deep learning. Nat Biomed Eng. 2018;2(3):158-164. doi:10.1038/s41551-018-0195-0

138 Yun JS, Kim J, Jung SH, et al. A deep learning model for screening type 2 diabetes from retinal photographs. Nutr Metab Cardiovasc Dis. 2022;32(5):1218-1226. doi:10.1016/j.numecd.2022.01.010

139 Korot E, Pontikos N, Liu X, et al. Predicting sex from retinal fundus photographs using automated deep learning. Sci Rep. 2021;11(1):10286. Published 2021 May 13. doi:10.1038/s41598-021-89743-x

140 Babenko B, Mitani A, Traynis I, et al. Detection of signs of disease in external photographs of the eyes via deep learning [published online ahead of print, 2022 Mar 29]. Nat Biomed Eng. 2022;1-14. doi:10.1038/s41551-022-00867-5

141 Allison K, Patel D, Alabi O. Epidemiology of Glaucoma: The Past, Present, and Predictions for the Future. Cureus. 2020;12(11):e11686. Published 2020 Nov 24. doi:10.7759/cureus.11686

142 von der Emde L, Pfau M, Holz FG, et al. AI-based structure-function correlation in age-related macular degeneration. Eye (Lond). 2021;35(8):2110-2118. doi:10.1038/s41433-021-01503-3

143 Linnehan R. Deep learning algorithm's prediction of RNFL thickness gauges risk for glaucoma conversion. Helio Ocular Surgery News. March 13, 2021. Accessed May 5, 2022. www.healio.com/news/ophthalmology/20210316/deep-learning-algorithms-prediction-of-rnfl-thickness-gauges-risk-for-glaucoma-conversion

144 Seeing Potential: How a team at Google is using AI to help doctors prevent blindness in diabetics. About Google. Accessed May 5, 2022. https://about.google/intl/ALL_us/stories/seeingpotential/

145 FDA permits marketing of artificial intelligence-based device to detect certain diabetes-related eye problems. U.S. Food & Drug Administration. April 11, 2018. Accessed May 5, 2022. https://www.fda.gov/news-events/press-announcements/fda-permits-marketing-artificial-intelligence-based-device-detect-certain-diabetes-related-eye

146 Over one-third of Americans live in areas lacking mental health professionals. USAFacts. Updated July 14, 2021. Accessed May 5, 2022. https://usafacts.org/articles/over-one-third-of-americans-live-in-areas-lacking-mental-health-professionals/

147 New Study Shows 60 Percent of U.S. Counties Without a Single Psychiatrist. New American Economy. October 23, 2017. Accessed May 5, 2022. https://www.newamericaneconomy.org/press-release/new-study-shows-60-percent-of-u-s-counties-without-a-single-psychiatrist/

148 Mental Disorders Cost Society Billions in Unearned Income. National Institutes of Health. May 7, 2008. Accessed May 5, 2022. https://www.nih.gov/news-events/news-releases/mental-disorders-cost-society-billions-unearned-income

149 Garg P, Glick S. AI's Potential to Diagnose and Treat Mental Illness. Harvard Business Review. October 22, 2018. Accessed May 5, 2022. https://hbr.org/2018/10/ais-potential-to-diagnose-and-treat-mental-illness

150 Wittchen HU, Mühlig S, Beesdo K. Mental disorders in primary care. Dialogues Clin Neurosci. 2003;5(2):115-128. doi:10.31887/DCNS.2003.5.2/huwittchen

151 Graham S, Depp C, Lee EE, et al. Artificial Intelligence for Mental Health and Mental Illnesses: An Overview. Curr Psychiatry Rep. 2019;21(11):116. Published 2019 Nov 7. doi:10.1007/s11920-019-1094-0

152 Blease C, Locher C, Leon-Carlyle M, Doraiswamy M. Artificial intelligence and the future of psychiatry: Qualitative findings from a global physician survey. Digit Health. 2020;6:2055207620968355. Published 2020 Oct 27. doi:10.1177/2055207620968355

153 Risk Group, Feusner J. Machine Learning For Mental Health Diagnosis. Risk Group LLC. June 21, 2019. Accessed May 5, 2022. https://riskgroupllc.com/machine-learning-for-mental-health-diagnosis/

154 Kosecki D. Online therapy vs in-person: What you should know. CNET. August 13, 2019. Accessed May 5, 2022. https://www.cnet.com/health/online-vs-in-person-therapy-cost-confidentiality-accessibility-and-more/

155 Dwyer DB, Falkai P, Koutsouleris N. Machine Learning Approaches for Clinical Psychology and Psychiatry. Annu Rev Clin Psychol. 2018 May 7;14:91-118. doi: 10.1146/annurev-clinpsy-032816-045037

156 Dosovitsky G, Pineda BS, Jacobson NC, Chang C, Escoredo M, Bunge EL. Artificial Intelligence Chatbot for Depression: Descriptive Study of Usage. JMIR Form Res. 2020;4(11):e17065. Published 2020 Nov 13. doi:10.2196/17065

157 Taliaz D, Spinrad A, Barzilay R, et al. Optimizing prediction of response to antidepressant medications using machine learning and integrated genetic, clinical, and demographic data. Transl Psychiatry. 2021;11(1):381. Published 2021 Jul 8. doi:10.1038/s41398-021-01488-3

158 Insel T, Cuthbert B, Garvey M, et al. Research domain criteria (RDoC): toward a new classification framework for research on mental disorders. Am J Psychiatry. 2010;167:748–51.

159 Kessler RC, Hwang I, Hoffmire CA, et al. Developing a practical suicide risk prediction model for targeting high-risk patients in the Veterans Health Administration. Int J Methods Psychiatr Res. 2017;26(3):1–14.

160 Eichstaedt JC, Smith RJ, Merchant RM, et al. Facebook language predicts depression in medical records. Proc Natl Acad Sci U S A. 2018;115(44):11203-11208. doi:10.1073/pnas.1802331115

161 Eichstaedt JC, Schwartz HA, Kern ML, et al. Psychological language on Twitter predicts county-level heart disease mortality. Psychol Sci. 2015;26(2):159-169. doi:10.1177/0956797614557867

162 Lupkin S. What Your Tweets May Say About Your Heart Health. ABC News. January 22, 2015. Accessed May 5, 2022. https://abcnews. go.com/Health/tweets-heart-health/story?id=28403774

163 2021 National Veteran Suicide Prevention Annual Report FI-NAL. U.S. Department of Veterans Affairs. September 9, 2021. Accessed May 5, 2022. https://www.mentalhealth.va.gov/docs/ data-sheets/2021/2021-National-Veteran-Suicide-Preven-tion-Annual-Report-FINAL-9-8-21.pdf

164 Richman M. Crisis prevention: Study evaluates VA program that identifies Vets at highest risk for suicide. U.S. Department of Veterans Affairs. September 20, 2018. Accessed May 5, 2022. https://www.re-search.va.gov/currents/0918-Study-evaluates-VA-program-that-identi-fies-Vets-at-highest-risk-for-suicide.cfm

165 McCarthy JF, Bossarte RM, Katz IR, et al. Predictive Modeling and Concentration of the Risk of Suicide: Implications for Preventive Interventions in the US Department of Veterans Affairs. Am J Public Health. 2015;105(9):1935-1942. doi:10.2105/AJPH.2015.302737

166 Kim S, Lee HK, Lee K. Detecting suicidal risk using MMPI-2 based on machine learning algorithm. Sci Rep. 2021;11(1):15310. Published 2021 Jul 28. doi:10.1038/s41598-021-94839-5

167 Lucas GM, Rizzo A, Gratch J, Scherer S, Stratou G, Boberg J, Morency LP. Reporting Mental Health Symptoms: Breaking Down Barriers to Care with Virtual Human Interviewers. Front. Robot. AI, 12 October 2017 https://doi.org/10.3389/frobt.2017.00051

168 Murphy T. Clarification: Health Care-Artificial Intelligence story. ABC News. November 26, 2019. Accessed May 5, 2022.

169 Xi Y, Xu P. Global colorectal cancer burden in 2020 and projections to 2040. Transl Oncol. 2021;14(10):101174.

170 An Astounding 16.6 Million Colonoscopies are Performed Annually in The United States. iData Research. August 8, 2018. Accessed May 6, 2022. https://idataresearch.com/an-astounding-19-million-colonosco-pies-are-performed-annually-in-the-united-states/

171 Park SY, Sargent D, Spofford I, Vosburgh KG, A-Rahim Y. A colon

video analysis framework for polyp detection. IEEE Trans Biomed Eng. 2012;59(5):1408-1418. doi:10.1109/TBME.2012.2188397

172 Repici A, Badalamenti M, Maselli R, et al. Efficacy of Real-Time Computer-Aided Detection of Colorectal Neoplasia in a Randomized Trial. Gastroenterology. 2020;159(2):512-520.e7. doi:10.1053/j.gastro.2020.04.062

173 Ishiyama M, Kudo S, Misawa M, et al. ID: 3521790 Does artificial intelligence improve neoplasms detection rate for colonoscopy? – A single center pilot study. Gastrointest Endosc. 2021;93(6)Suppl:AB191-2. doi.org/10.1016/j.gie.2021.03.433.

174 Richter R, Burns J, et al. Artificial Intelligence Helps Keep Adenoma Detection Constant Over the Day. UEG Journal. 2021;9(8):MP 077

175 FDA Authorizes Marketing of First Device that Uses Artificial Intelligence to Help Detect Potential Signs of Colon Cancer. U.S. Food & Drug Administration. April 9, 2021. Accessed May 6, 2022. https://www.fda.gov/news-events/press-announcements/fda-authorizes-marketing-first-device-uses-artificial-intelligence-help-detect-potential-signs-colon

176 Rex DK, Kahi C, O'Brien M, et al. The American Society for Gastrointestinal Endoscopy PIVI (Preservation and Incorporation of Valuable Endoscopic Innovations) on real-time endoscopic assessment of the histology of diminutive colorectal polyps. Gastrointest Endosc. 2011;73(3):419-422. doi:10.1016/j.gie.2011.01.023

177 Rodriguez-Diaz E, Jepeal LI, Baffy G, et al. Artificial Intelligence-Based Assessment of Colorectal Polyp Histology by Elastic-Scattering Spectroscopy. Dig Dis Sci. 2022;67(2):613-621. doi:10.1007/s10620-021-06901-x

178 Komeda Y, Handa H, Matsui R, et al. Artificial intelligence-based endoscopic diagnosis of colorectal polyps using residual networks. PLoS One. 2021;16(6):e0253585. Published 2021 Jun 22. doi:10.1371/journal.pone.0253585

179 Visaggi P, Barberio B, Gregori D, et al. Systematic review with meta-analysis: artificial intelligence in the diagnosis of oesophageal diseases. Aliment Pharmacol Ther. 2022;55(5):528-540. doi:10.1111/apt.16778

180 Then EO, Lopez M, Saleem S, et al. Esophageal Cancer: An Updated

Surveillance Epidemiology and End Results Database Analysis. World J Oncol. 2020;11(2):55-64. doi:10.14740/wjon1254

181 Zhang SM, Wang YJ, Zhang ST. Accuracy of artificial intelligence-assisted detection of esophageal cancer and neoplasms on endoscopic images: A systematic review and meta-analysis. J Dig Dis. 2021;22(6):318-328. doi:10.1111/1751-2980.12992

182 Fernandes SR, Pinto JSLD, Marques da Costa P, Correia L; GEDII. Disagreement Among Gastroenterologists Using the Mayo and Rutgeerts Endoscopic Scores. Inflamm Bowel Dis. 2018;24(2):254-260. doi:10.1093/ibd/izx066

183 Maeda Y, Kudo SE, Mori Y, et al. Fully automated diagnostic system with artificial intelligence using endocytoscopy to identify the presence of histologic inflammation associated with ulcerative colitis (with video). Gastrointest Endosc. 2019;89(2):408-415. doi:10.1016/j.gie.2018.09.024

184 Maeda Y, Kudo SE, Ogata N, et al. Evaluation in real-time use of artificial intelligence during colonoscopy to predict relapse of ulcerative colitis: A prospective study. Gastrointest Endosc. 2022;95(4):747-756. e2. doi:10.1016/j.gie.2021.10.019

185 Plevy S, Silverberg MS, Lockton S, et al. Combined serological, genetic, and inflammatory markers differentiate non-IBD, Crohn's disease, and ulcerative colitis patients. Inflamm Bowel Dis. 2013;19(6):1139-1148. doi:10.1097/MIB.0b013e318280b19e

186 Stidham RW, Takenaka K. Artificial Intelligence for Disease Assessment in Inflammatory Bowel Disease: How Will it Change Our Practice? Gastroenterology. 2022;162(5):1493-1506. doi:10.1053/j.gastro.2021.12.238

187 Keogan MT, Lo JY, Freed KS, et al. Outcome analysis of patients with acute pancreatitis by using an artificial neural network. Acad Radiol. 2002;9(4):410-419. doi:10.1016/s1076-6332(03)80186-1

188 Kenner B, Chari ST, Kelsen D, et al. Artificial Intelligence and Early Detection of Pancreatic Cancer: 2020 Summative Review. Pancreas. 2021;50(3):251-279. doi:10.1097/MPA.0000000000001762

189 Mukherjee S, Patra A, Khasawneh H, Korfiatis P, et al. Radiomics-Based Machine-Learning Models Can Detect Pancreatic Cancer on Prediagnostic CTs at a Substantial Lead Time Prior to Clinical

Diagnosis. Gastroenterology. 2022 Jul 1:S0016-5085(22)00728-4. doi: 10.1053/j.gastro.2022.06.066. Epub ahead of print. PMID: 35788343.

190 Ahn JC, Attia ZI, Rattan P, et al. Development of the AI-Cirrhosis-ECG Score: An Electrocardiogram-Based Deep Learning Model in Cirrhosis. Am J Gastroenterol. 2022;117(3):424-432. doi:10.14309/ajg.0000000000001617

191 Bosworth T. AI Generates an Accurate Technique For Detection of Cirrhosis. Gastroenterology & Endoscopy News. November 2, 2021. Accessed May 6, 2022. https://www.gastroendonews.com/Hepatology-in-Focus/Article/04-19/AI-Generates-For-Detection-of-Cirrhosis/64812

192 Lane T. A short history of robotic surgery. Ann R Coll Surg Engl. 2018;100(6_sup):5-7. doi:10.1308/rcsann.supp1.5

193 Kalan S, Chauhan S, Coelho RF, et al. History of robotic surgery. J Robot Surg. 2010;4(3):141-147. doi:10.1007/s11701-010-0202-2

194 Sorokin I, Sundaram V, Singla N, et al. Robot-Assisted Versus Open Simple Prostatectomy for Benign Prostatic Hyperplasia in Large Glands: A Propensity Score-Matched Comparison of Perioperative and Short-Term Outcomes. J Endourol. 2017;31(11):1164-1169. doi:10.1089/end.2017.0489

195 Bindal V, Bhatia P, Dudeja U, et al. Review of contemporary role of robotics in bariatric surgery. J Minim Access Surg. 2015;11(1):16-21. doi:10.4103/0972-9941.147673

196 Orady M, Hrynewych A, Nawfal AK, Wegienka G. Comparison of robotic-assisted hysterectomy to other minimally invasive approaches. JSLS. 2012;16(4):542-548. doi:10.4293/108680812X13462882736899

197 Weinberg L, Rao S, Escobar PF. Robotic surgery in gynecology: an updated systematic review. Obstet Gynecol Int. 2011;2011:852061. doi:10.1155/2011/852061

198 Yanagawa F, Perez M, Bell T, Grim R, Martin J, Ahuja V. Critical Outcomes in Nonrobotic vs Robotic-Assisted Cardiac Surgery. JAMA Surg. 2015;150(8):771-777. doi:10.1001/jamasurg.2015.1098

199 Writing Committee Members, Lawton JS, Tamis-Holland JE, et al. 2021 ACC/AHA/SCAI Guideline for Coronary Artery Revascularization: A Report of the American College of Cardiology/American Heart Association Joint Committee on Clinical Practice

Guidelines [published correction appears in J Am Coll Cardiol. 2022 Apr 19;79(15):1547]. J Am Coll Cardiol. 2022;79(2):e21-e129. doi:10.1016/j.jacc.2021.09.006

200 Tsui C, Klein R, Garabrant M. Minimally invasive surgery: national trends in adoption and future directions for hospital strategy. Surg Endosc. 2013;27(7):2253-2257. doi:10.1007/s00464-013-2973-9

201 Gottlieb S. Surgeons perform transatlantic operation using fibreoptics. BMJ. 2001;323(7315):713.

202 Alemzadeh H, Raman J, Leveson N, Kalbarczyk Z, Iyer RK. Adverse Events in Robotic Surgery: A Retrospective Study of 14 Years of FDA Data. PLoS One. 2016;11(4):e0151470. Published 2016 Apr 20. doi:10.1371/journal.pone.0151470

203 Collier M, Fu R. AI: Healthcare's new nervous system. accenture health. July 30, 2020. Accessed May 6, 2022. https://www.accenture.com/au-en/insights/health/artificial-intelligence-healthcare

204 Obermeyer Z, Powers B, Vogeli C, Mullainathan S. Dissecting racial bias in an algorithm used to manage the health of populations. Science. 2019;366(6464):447-453. doi:10.1126/science.aax2342

205 Hardesty L. Study finds gender and skin-type bias in commercial artificial-intelligence systems. MIT News. Massachusetts Institute of Technology. February 11, 2018. Accessed May 6, 2022. https://news.mit.edu/2018/study-finds-gender-skin-type-bias-artificial-intelligence-systems-0212

206 DeepMind faces legal action over NHS data use. BBC News. October 1, 2021. Accessed May 6, 2022. https://www.bbc.com/news/technology-58761324

207 Wong A, Otles E, Donnelly JP, et al. External Validation of a Widely Implemented Proprietary Sepsis Prediction Model in Hospitalized Patients [published correction appears in JAMA Intern Med. 2021 Aug 1;181(8):1144]. JAMA Intern Med. 2021;181(8):1065-1070. doi:10.1001/jamainternmed.2021.2626

208 Stanford Medicine. Katherine Chou, Google – Stanford Medicine Big Data | Precision Health 2018. Youtube. June 21, 2018. Accessed May 6, 2022. https://www.youtube.com/watch?v=bQunKHZywOc

209 The Lancet Commission on Diagnostics. Accessed August 25, 2022. https://diagnosticscommission.org/

210 Si M, Yu C. Chinese robot becomes world's first machine to pass medical exam. China Daily. Updated November 10, 2017. Accessed May 7, 2022. http://www.chinadaily.com.cn/bizchina/tech/2017-11/10/content_34362656.htm